Aids to Undergraduate Obstetrics and Gynaecology

Aids to Undergraduate Obstetrics and Gynaecology

Christopher Sinclair

MB BS BSc

Senior House Officer in Obstetrics,
Northwick Park Hospital,
London

J. Beverley Webb

FRCS MRCOG

Senior Registrar,
Hammersmith Hospital,
London

CHURCHILL LIVINGSTONE
EDINBURGH LONDON MELBOURNE AND NEW YORK 1986

CHURCHILL LIVINGSTONE
Medical Division of Longman Group Limited

Distributed in the United States of America by
Churchill Livingstone Inc., 1560 Broadway, New
York, N.Y. 10036, and by associated companies,
branches and representatives throughout the
world.

First published 1986

ISBN 0 443 03025 1

British Library Cataloguing in Publication Data
Sinclair, Christopher C. R.
   Aids to undergraduate obstetrics and gynaecology.
   1. Gynecology   2. Obstetrics
   I. Title   II. Webb, J. Beverley
   618   RG101
   ISBN 0-443-03025-1

Library of Congress Cataloging in Publication Data
Sinclair, Christopher C. R.
   Aids to undergraduate obstetrics and gynaecology.
   Includes index.
   1. Gynecology — Outlines, syllabi, etc.   2. Obstetrics
— Outlines, syllabi, etc.   I. Webb, J. Beverley.
II. Title.   [DNLM: 1. Gynecology — outlines.   2. Obstetrics
— outlines.   WP 18 S616a]
RG112.S56   1985   618'.02'02   85-5958
ISBN 0-443-03025-1

Produced by Longman Singapore Publishers (Pte) Ltd.
Printed in Singapore.

Preface

This book is intended to enable the undergraduate to revise quickly and easily, by means of lists, the subject of Obstetrics and Gynaecology. The lists will jog the memory and aid recall of the detail relating to the subject under revision. It is hoped that this will be of benefit in preparing for MCQs and written examinations. In addition some of the lists will provide ready-made essay plans.

The authors believe that examination technique is as important as adequate factual knowledge. When writing an essay a plan must be constructed, and time left at the end for reading through and correction, and the underlining of important points which the candidate wishes to highlight to the examiner. The plans may be drawn up singly as each essay is tackled, or the first part of the examination may be allotted to planning all the essays, but whichever system is adopted, accurate time-keeping throughout is essential. It is worth noting that the candidate will often find that while preparing the second plan, ideas for the first will enter the mind, and that while writing the first essay, ideas for the last plan will interrupt the planned flow of thought. For this reason the second system is usually better.

We have not suggested a reading list or provided references since most undergraduates find their own books with a style that suits them. Nonetheless, we encourage the student to research further any points encountered with which he/she is not familiar, and more importantly, get to know the practices and their rationale in your teaching hospital. This will give you the ability and confidence to discuss them in a viva where you may well encounter external examiners who hold differing views to those you have been taught, e.g. the induction of labour. Do not worry; the internal examiner is there to see fair play and all that is expected of you is to prove that you are safe to be allowed to practice. Provided you achieve this, there is no reason why you should not succeed in passing your final examinations.

London, 1986

Acknowledgements

The authors would like to express their gratitude to Mrs Joyce Webb and Miss Julie Pollicott for typing the manuscripts, and to Churchill Livingstone for their tolerant and helpful guidance in the preparation of this book.

Contents

Contents

PART 1

Reproductive anatomy and physiology

Reproductive anatomy and physiology

This chapter outlines key anatomical and physiological facts, knowledge of which simplifies the understanding of clinical obstetrics and gynaecology. The selection has been made partly on the basis of clinical relevance and partly on the degree of interest shown in the matter by examiners.

MATERNAL AND GYNAECOLOGICAL ANATOMY

The bony pelvis
The bony pelvis provides the basic framework of the birth canal: for this reason its shape, size and clinically identifiable landmarks should be understood.

The pelvic diameters
In the past cephalo-pelvic disproportion (disparity between the size and shape of the fetal head and the maternal birth canal) accounted for a large proportion of difficult and obstructed labours. This resulted in the obstetrician's classical interest in pelvic dimensions. Figure 1 defines the key diameters.

Note that there is a 'pattern' to these measurements.

Pelvic Shape
The pelvic inlet (brim) is bean-shaped with its greatest diameter placed transversely: hence the antero-posterior (AP) diameter of the fetal head usually enters the pelvis in the transverse diameter.

The mid-cavity is roughly cylindrical to allow rotation of the presenting part and shoulders, and in breech presentations, the after-coming head.

The outlet is diagonally shaped with its greatest diameter placed anterio-posteriorly: the fetal head therefore prefers to leave the pelvis in the AP diameter. The axis of the outlet is at 90° to the axis of the inlet.

3

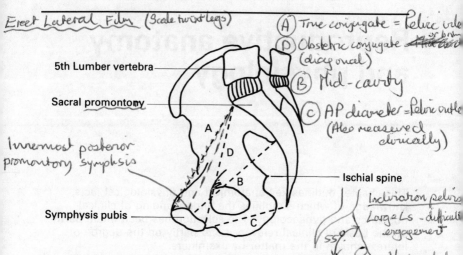

Erect Lateral Film (Scale twixt legs)

(A) True conjugate = Pelvic inlet
(D) Obstetric conjugate = + or brim
    (diagonal)
(B) Mid-cavity
(C) AP diameter = Pelvic outlet
    (Also measured clinically)

5th Lumber vertebra

Sacral promontory

Innermost posterior promontory symphysis

Symphysis pubis

Ischial spine

Inclination pelvis
Large Ls - difficult engagement

55°

Horizontal

Fig. 1 Side view of the bony pelvis showing key diameters: for typical measurements see Table 1. A = pelvic inlet (brim); B = mid-cavity; C = pelvic outlet; D = diagonal (obstetric) conjugate

Shortest AP diameter of pelvic inlet = Obstetric conjugate

Table 1. Average dimensions of the bony pelvis (cm)

	Anterioposterior	Oblique	Transverse
Inlet	11	12	13
Midcavity	12	12	12
Outlet	13	12	11

The rotation of the fetal head during its passage through the pelvis is one of the key events in labour: failure to rotate, for example, may result in 'deep transverse arrest'.

Pelvic Landmarks

Sacral promontory: palpation of this on vaginal examination suggests a short diagonal (obstetric) conjugate and therefore a small pelvis.

Ischial spines: these provide useful landmarks on the side of the birth canal to assess the descent of the presenting part.

Pubic arch: this provides a crude assessment of pelvic outlet dimensions.

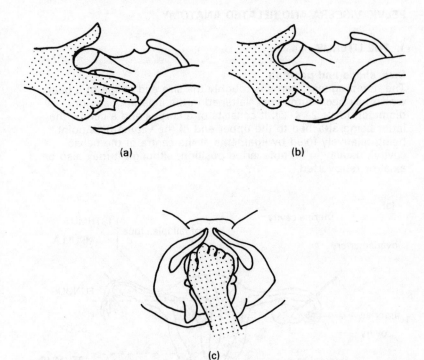

Fig. 2 (a) Attempting to palpate the sacral promontory; (b) palpating the ischial spine; (c) assessment of the intertuberous diameter

The method of palpating these landmarks is shown in figure 2.

The pelvic floor
The pelvic floor (or diaphragm) is composed of muscles and condensations of fascia, perforated in three places by the urethra, vagina and anus. It performs a number of important functions including:
1. Support of the pelvic (and abdominal) viscera.
2. Maintenance of continence (urinary and faecal).
3. Assisting in the rotation of the fetal head during labour.

It may be damaged in labour and subsequently fail to perform its functions, especially those of support and the maintenance of continence.

PELVIC VISCERA AND RELATED ANATOMY

1. THE UTERUS

Size, shape and position

The non-pregnant uterus is roughly the size and shape of a pear which has been somewhat flattened in the anterio-posterior diameter, (3″ × 2″ × 1″). It consists of a corpus and a cervix, the latter being attached to the upper end of the vagina (this point being relatively fixed by ligaments at the centre of the pelvic cavity), usually in an anteverted position, although it may also be axial or retroverted.

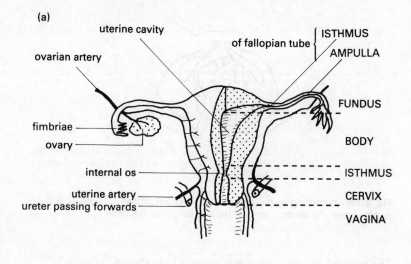

(a)

uterine cavity
ovarian artery
{ ISTHMUS / AMPULLA } of fallopian tube
fimbriae
ovary
internal os
uterine artery
ureter passing forwards

FUNDUS
BODY
ISTHMUS
CERVIX
VAGINA

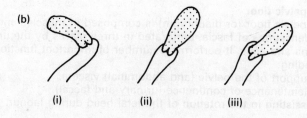

(b)

(i)   (ii)   (iii)

Fig. 3 (a) Anatomy of the uterus and (b) orientation of the uterus in (i) anteversion; (ii) axial position and (iii) retroversion

During pregnancy the uterus undergoes massive enlargement, becoming palpable abdominally at about 12–14 weeks gestation; thereafter it continues to grow as shown.

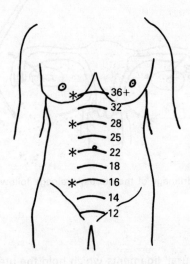

Fig. 4 Usual height of the uterine fundus at different weeks of gestation. Those levels marked * represent key dates which can usefully be learnt to allow extrapolation to other dates

Blood supply and lymphatics

Blood supply: mainly from the uterine artery which arises from the internal iliac artery, and subsequently anastomases with the ovarian artery in the broad ligament. Just before reaching the uterus (at the level of the internal os) it crosses over the ureter, so exposing the latter to risk at hysterectomy. (Aide memoire: water under bridge).

Lymphatics: clinically highly relevant because of metastatic spread from carcinoma. Note that the main drainage channels for the uterine body and uterine cervix follow different routes (the respective carcinomas also differ in their propensity to lymphatic spread).

Volsellum

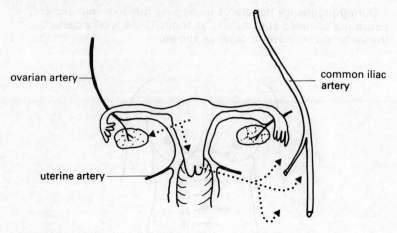

ovarian artery

common iliac artery

uterine artery

Fig. 5 Lymphatic drainage of the uterus; drainage follows the direction of the dotted lines.

Ligaments

The main 'structural' ligaments which hold the uterus in place are attached to the cervix, from which they radiate out to become attached to various structures as shown in figure 6.

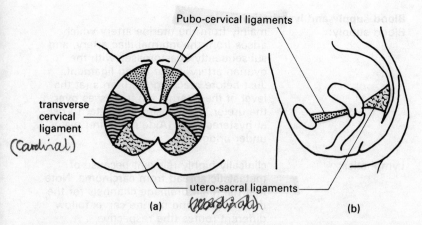

Pubo-cervical ligaments

transverse cervical ligament

(Cardinal)

utero-sacral ligaments

(a)   (b)

Fig. 6 The ligaments of the uterine cervix (a) as seen from below and (b) lateral view

The broad ligament

This is not a true ligament but a fold of peritoneum draped over the fallopian tubes stretching from the lateral wall of the uterus to the side walls of the pelvis. (Anteriorly the peritoneum sweeps off the anterior uterus over the bladder forming the utero-vesical pouch. Posteriorly the peritoneum sweeps down the back of the uterus, cervix and posterior fornix of the vagina onto the anterior rectum forming the Pouch of Douglas.)

The round ligament

Represents the remains of the lower part of the gubernaculum and passes from the upper outer corner of the uterus to the internal inguinal ring, and from there to the labium majora. It is composed of smooth muscle and is greatly stretched in pregnancy which may give rise to pain.

Congenital uterine anomalies

Four of the more common anomalies are illustrated. Associated urinary tract abnormalities are common and therefore IVU is essential.

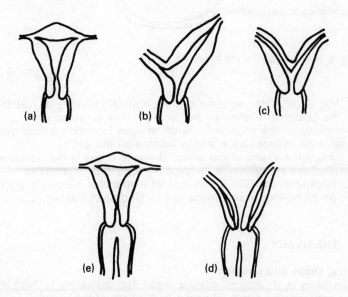

Fig. 7 Common congenital uterine anomalies. (a) Normal arrangement; (b) rudimentary horn; (c) bicornuate uterus, normal vagina; (d) normal uterus with vaginal septum; (e) bicornuate uterus with septate vagina

Histology

The body of the uterus is lined internally by the endometrium, the innermost layer of which consists of columnar epithelium, which is invaginated to form the uterine glands. For this reason adenocarcinoma is the commonest endometrial carcinoma.

The cervical canal is lined internally with secretory columnar epithelium, whilst the vaginal portion is covered by squamous epithelium.

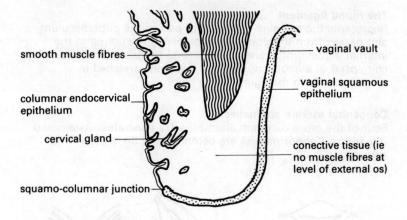

smooth muscle fibres

columnar endocervical epithelium

cervical gland

squamo-columnar junction

vaginal vault

vaginal squamous epithelium

conective tissue (ie no muscle fibres at level of external os)

Fig. 8 Histology of the uterine cervix

'Migration' of the squamo-columnar junction outwards results in the columnar epithelium becoming visible on speculum examination: the so-called cervical erosion (common before the age of 20, in pregnancy, and in women on the 'pill').

Carcinoma-in-situ of the cervix normally arises in the transition zone where epithelium is undergoing squamous metaplasia. Carcinoma-in-situ (CIN 3: cervical intra-epithelial neoplasia 3) may go on to develop a squamous cell carcinoma of the cervix.

2. THE OVARY

Size, shape and position

The ovary is an almond shaped organ approximately $1\frac{1}{2}''$ long in the reproductive years, attached to the back of the broad ligament by the mesovarium. It is attached to the uterus by the round ligament of the ovary, which represents the remains of the upper half of the gubernaculum.

Blood supply and lymphatics

Blood supply: the ovary is supplied by the ovarian artery which (for embryological reasons) arises from the aorta at the level of the renal arteries.

Lymphatics: mainly to the para-aortic nodes, along the course of the ovarian arteries, but also to the uterine fundus, and so to the contralateral ovary.

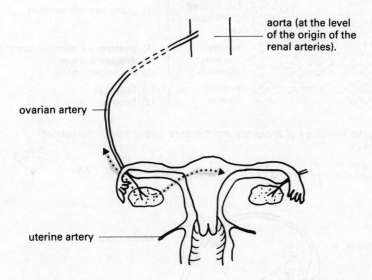

aorta (at the level of the origin of the renal arteries).

ovarian artery

uterine artery

Fig. 9 Lymphatic drainage of the ovaries; drainage follows the direction of the dotted lines

Histology

The histology of the ovary provides one of the few ways of rationalising neoplastic tumours by cell of origin (see figure 10).

3. FETAL ANATOMY

Although the fetal shoulders represent its widest part, they seldom cause problems in labour and in practice it is the fetal head that matters. The various parts and diameters are shown in figure 11.

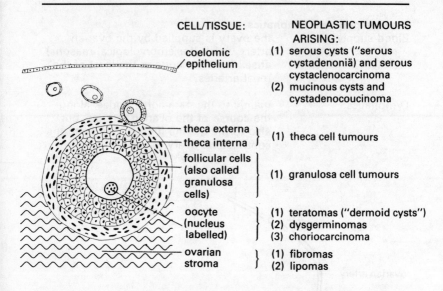

CELL/TISSUE:	NEOPLASTIC TUMOURS ARISING:
coelomic epithelium	(1) serous cysts ("serous cystadenoniä) and serous cystaclenocarcinoma
	(2) mucinous cysts and cystadenocoucinoma
theca externa theca interna }	(1) theca cell tumours
follicular cells (also called granulosa cells)	(1) granulosa cell tumours
oocyte (nucleus labelled)	(1) teratomas ("dermoid cysts")
	(2) dysgerminomas
	(3) choriocarcinoma
ovarian stroma	(1) fibromas
	(2) lipomas

Fig. 10 Histology of the ovary and tumours arising from different cell types

Posterior fontanelle is the TRIANGULAR ONE

occiput

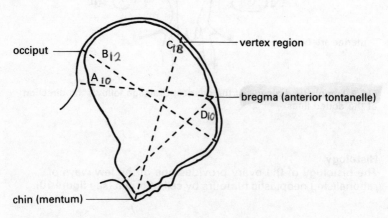

occiput — B 12   C 18 — vertex region
A 10
D 10 — bregma (anterior tontanelle)
chin (mentum)

Fig. 11 Parts of the fetal head and the important diameters of the fetal head; for explanation of diameters A-D see Table 2

Table 2: Fetal head diameters (*measurements in cm*)

Diameter	Presentation	Name of diameter	Average size (cm)
A	Vertex	Suboccipito-bregmatic	10
B	Poorly flexed Vertex	Occipito-frontal	12
C	Brow	Mento-vertical	13
D	Face	Submento-bregmatic	10

Note that the degree of flexion of the fetal head in relation to the fetal neck will define its presentation, and so the presenting diameter. The normal presentation is by the vertex, but others occur.

The fetal head is said to be engaged when its greatest diameter has passed through the pelvic inlet. Since this is assumed to be the smallest pelvic diameter, it is implied that once the head is engaged the labour will not become obstructed.

4. PLACENTAL ANATOMY

The placenta is a disc of tissue made up of approximately 20 cotyledons. The cord normally enters it roughly in the centre. Various placental anomalies exist including:

Battledora placenta: cord enters the placenta at the side (marginal insertion).

Velamentous insertion: the umbilical vessels run in the membranes before entering the placenta.

Bipartite placenta: the placenta is divided into two separate lobes, joined by vessels running in the membranes.

Succentiurate placenta: an accessory separate cotyledon is joined to the main placenta by vessels running in the membranes.

These anomalies may result in:

Accidental damage to the umbilical vessels at the time of membrane rupture.

Accidental retention of products of conception when the placenta consists of two or more parts.

5. PHYSIOLOGY

The menstrual cycle

An understanding of the menstrual cycle is essential to the understanding of gynaecological endocrinology. The events that make up the cycle are as follows:

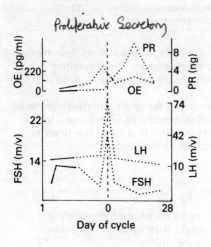

(a) early follicular phase: Low oestrogen and progesterone levels cause positive feedback stimulation secretion of FSH (and LH), levels of which therefore rise: the increased FSH level stimulates follicular development (but note FSH does not *initiate* follicular development).

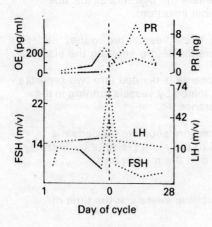

(b) late follicular phase: As the developing follicle matures, it secretes increasing amounts of oestrogen, which at the initially lower concentrations causes negative feedback inhibition of FSH, levels of which therefore fall.

Figure 12: The Menstrual Cycle: OE = oestrogen; PR = progesterone; FSH = follicle stimulating hormone; LH = lutenizing hormone; O = LH surge: ovulation occurs approximately 12 hours later

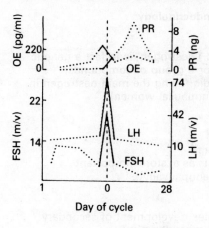

(c) LH surge and ovulation:
At higher levels, oestrogen causes positive feedback stimulation of LH secretion, resulting in the LH surge, and, 12 hours later, ovulation

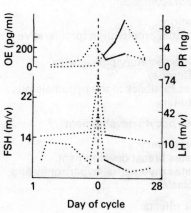

Secretory

(d) early luteal phase:
Oestrogen levels decrease initially, probably due to follicular disruption; the corpus luteum then starts to secrete increasing amounts of progesterone (and some oestrogen) and FSH and LH levels drop due to negative feedback inhibition, so preventing any further follicular development.

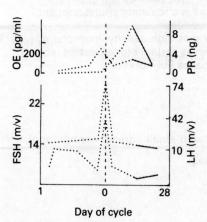

(e) late luteal phase:
In the event of no pregnancy, the corpus luteum fails and progesterone levels drop, so removing the negative feedback inhibition of FSH (and LH), levels of which therefore start to rise, so stimulating the development of a new follicle (but not initiating follicular development).

Obstetric and gynaecological endocrinology

Oestrogen

Chemical nature: steroid ('oestrogen' is in fact a generic term for a group of compounds: oestradiol being the main oestrogen in premenopausal women).

Produced by: Ovary.
Placenta.
(Fat acts as a 'store' [important postmenopausally]).

Actions: — Promotes development of secondary sexual characteristics.

Menstruation:
endometrial proliferation (proliferative phase)
promotes secretory phase (with progesterone)
provides feedback to the hypothalamus and pituitary

— Stimulates oocyte development.

— During pregnancy:
stimulates breast development
stimulates myometrial hypertrophy and hyperplasia

— Metabolic effects:
encourages calcification of bone
increases circulating cholesterol and triglycerides
decreases high density lipoproteins (HDLs)
increases certain blood clotting factors
decreases fibrinolysis.

Progesterone

Chemical nature: Steroid.

Produced by: Ovary (with small adrenal contribution).

Placenta.

Actions: (requires oestrogen to work)
    Causes changes in vaginal epithelium.
    Cervical mucus decreases in amount and becomes thicker.
    Promotes secretory changes in endometrium.
    Raises uterine excitation threshold.
    Generalised smooth muscle relaxation.
    Stimulates glandular development in breast.
    Metabolic effects — generally catabolic.

Human placental lactogen
Chemical nature: Protein (similar to growth hormone and
                        prolactin).

Secreted by: The placenta. Level rises during
                        pregnancy and then plateaus at 35 weeks.

Actions: ? alters carbohydrate metabolism.
                        Pregnancy can apparently progress
                        normally without it.

Human chorionic gonadotrophin
Chemical nature: Protein (similar to pituitary LH)

Secreted by: The placenta level peaks at 12 weeks and
                        then falls off.

Actions: Early — prolongs corpus luteum.
                        Late — ? controls progesterone
                        metabolism.

Follicle stimulating hormone (FSH)
Chemical nature: Glycoprotein.

Secreted by: Pituitary under control of GnRH (q.v.).

Actions: Stimulates follicular growth (but does
                        not initiate it).

Luteinising hormone (LH)
Chemical nature: Glycoprotein.

Secreted by: Pituitary under control of GnRH (q.v.).

Actions: Stimulates ovulation.
                        Follicular steroidogenesis.
                        Follicular maturation and rupture.
                        Luteinises the corpus luteum.

Prolactin

Chemical nature:	Polypeptide.
Secreted by:	Pituitary.
Actions:	Initially stimulates milk secretion. High levels inhibit ovarian oestrogen secretion.

Gonadotrophin releasing hormone (GnRH)

Chemical nature:	Decapeptide.
Secreted by:	The hypothalamus.
Actions:	Stimulates FSH and LH secretion.

Landmarks in Fetal Development

2–3 days post-conception:	Implantation.
3–4 weeks post-conception:	Heart starts to beat (detectable by ultrasound scan from 6 weeks *gestation*).
8 weeks:	Majority of organ development has occured and further development is by growth.
16 weeks (multigravidas) 18 weeks (primigravidas):	Quickening (mother first notices fetal movements).
Approximately 26 weeks:	Fetal heart beat first detectable clinically (i.e. by fetal stethoscope).
32 weeks:	Fetal outcome as good as at term in special centres.
34 weeks:	Surfactant production starts to rise.
38 weeks+:	Term (i.e. delivery at this time carries minimum perinatal risk).
40 weeks+:	*Post term.*

PART 2

Gynaecology

Gynaecological symptomatology

GYNAECOLOGICAL SYMPTOMATOLOGY

Menstrual disturbances — see p. 28.
Urological disorders — see p. 67.

Both in clinical practice and in examinations the question frequently arises as to what pathology may be responsible for particular symptoms. Usually this information can only be presented in bare list form, but below an attempt is made to present these lists in the most rational manner, a system which it is hoped may aid recall.

As a general rule it is better to learn broad headings before specific causes, partly because this provides a rational route of recall, and partly because it avoids concentrating on obscure and unimportant causes of a certain condition.

DYSPAREUNIA

Definition: Painful and/or difficult sexual intercourse

Classifications: (Onset)
  — Primary — always been present
  — Secondary — acquired after previous painfree intercourse

  (Anatomical)
  — Superficial — felt at or around introitus
  — Deep — felt deep in pelvis

Superficial dyspareunia

Most commonly due to thrush. Post episiotomy discomfort is also common and almost always settles without plastic surgery.

Causes: (1) Psychological/vaginisimus (=spasm of Levator ani: controversial) /Poor lubrication
(2) Infections/inflammations of the vulva and vagina:
— Candida

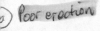 Poor erection

21

— Infected sebaceous cyst
- Trichomonas vaginalis
- Bartholin's cyst/abscess   Irritant chemical
- Atrophic vaginitis
- Vulval dystrophies.

(3) Local lesions causing vaginal narrowing:
   Post episiotomy scarring
   Other vaginal surgery

(4) Rare congenital abnormalities, e.g.
   vaginal septum, absent vagina

(5) Imperforate hymen

Deep dyspareunia

Causes:

? Type of pain
? Duration "
? Only on thrusting

(1) Pelvic inflammatory disease — acute and
   chronic (including cervicitis)
(2) Endometriosis
(3) Pelvic tumours
(4) Ectopic pregnancy
(5) Loaded sigmoid colon
(6) Possibly retroverted uterus and/or
   prolapse ovaries (opinions vary) — so-
   called 'collision dyspareunia'.
(7) Psychosexual disorders should not be
   forgotten: psychiatric opinion prior to
   surgery may be wise.

DYSMENORRHOEA

Definition:

Painful menstruation (some might add
'sufficient to cause inconvenience to the
patient' since most women have some
degree of discomfort associated with
their periods).

Classification:

Primary dysmenorrhoea (idiopathic,
intrinsic, spasmodic dysmenorrhoea):
   Patient is usually nulliparous.
   Pain starts with flow of menses, and
      disappears within 1–2 days.
   Low crampy midline pain, often
      associated with autonomic nervous
      system disturbance — nausea,
      vomiting and diarrhoea.
   Probably due to release of
      prostaglandins into circulation at time
      of menstruation.
   Not associated with other
      gynaecological pathology.

Secondary *dysmenorrhoea* (acquired,
extrinsic, congestive dysmenorrhoea):
  Pain begins up to 5 days premenstrually
    and reaches a peak either with
    commencement of menstruation or
    with peak of flow, settling soon
    afterwards.
  Constant (as opposed to crampy) pain,
    often lateralised to one side.
  Patient is usually over 20 years old.
  Usually associated with an secondary to
    organic pelvic pathology, e.g.
    endometriosis, pelvic inflammatory
    disease.

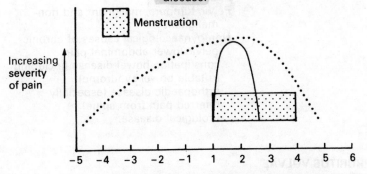

**Day of menstrual cycle (negative numbers
indicate number of days preceding start of flow)**

Fig. 13 Relationship of pain to menstrual flow in primary dysmenorrhoea
(solid line) and secondary dysmenorrhoea (dotted line)

PELVIC PAIN

Acute pelvic pain
Causes:
  1. All the causes of chronic pelvic pain (q.v.).
  2. Associated with pregnancy:
       ectopic pregnancy
       abortion
  3. Complications of ovarian cysts, e.g.
       torsion, haemorrhage, corpus luteum
       rupture.
  4. Dysmenorrhoea (q.v.)
  5. Infections and inflammations (especially
       gonorrhoea) — 'pelvic inflammatory
       disease'.

(6) Complications of fibroids, e.g. red
   degeneration of pregnancy. *or pill*
(7) Uterine contractions in trying to expel
   items from uterine cavity, e.g. polyp,
   intra-uterine contraceptive device.
(8) Mittelschmerz (q.v.)
(9) Non-gynaecological causes of acute
   pelvic/lower abdominal pain, e.g.
   appendicitis, diverticulitis, cystitis.

Chronic Pelvic Pain
Causes: (1) Infections — 'chronic pelvic
                       inflammatory disease'.
                   (2) Endometriosis
                   (3) Pelvic tumours, malignant and non-
                       malignant
                   (4) Non-gynaecological causes of chronic
                       pelvic/lower abdominal pain:
                       constipation/bowel disease (including
                       irritable bowel syndrome)
                       orthopaedic disease (especially
                       referred pain from spine)
                       urological disease.

PRURITUS VULVAE

Ninety per cent of cases in practice are thrush. Always exclude
diabetes.

Definition: Itching of the vulva, generally taken to
                     include the perineal skin.

Causes: (1) Irritation secondary to vaginal discharge
                       (q.v.).
                   (2) Vulval infections — bacterial, fungal,
                       viral (NB Herpes genitalis is usually
                       painful).
                   (3) Vulval infestations, e.g. lice, scabies.
                   (4) Bartholin's gland cyst/abscess (usually
                       are painless/painful though).
                   (5) Neoplasms — vulval, vaginal (often
                       symptomless unless they bleed).
                   (6) Vulval dystrophies, atrophic and
                       hypertrophic.
                   (7) Urological disease, e.g. incontinence.
                   (8) Dermatological disorders which happen
                       to affect vulva.

(9) Systemic disease causing general or
    local pruritus, e.g. diabetes mellitus (±
    associated fungal infection), liver
    disease, uraemia.
(10) Local (anal) disease, e.g. piles.
(11) Psychosomatic

VAGINAL DISCHARGE

Classification:

(1) Normal — non-offensive, clear mucoid
    discharge, heavier mid-cycle at
    ovulation.
(2) Cervicitis — milky viscoid.
(3) Vaginal infections:
    candida — white, curdlike
(4) Trichomonas vaginalis — frothy,
    yellow-green
(5) Pyogenic — foul-smelling, brown,
    watery.
(6) Neoplasms, e.g. uterine, cervical, vaginal
    — foul-smelling, brown, watery (often
    associated with infection).
(7) Foreign bodies (common cause of
    discharge in pre-pubertal age group).
(8) Fistulae — urinary and faecal.
(9) Miscellaneous (non-pathological) —
    semen, douches, pessaries.

GALACTORRHOEA

Definition: Inappropriate, non-puerperal lactation.

Causes:

(1) Prolactin secreting pituitary tumours.
(2) Drugs, e.g. phenothiazines, oral
    contraceptive pill, methyldopa.
(3) Ectopic prolactin secretion, e.g.
    bronchogenic carcinoma.
(4) Hypothalamic lesion/pituitary stalk
    section.
(5) Hypothyroidism

MITTELSCHMERZ

Definition: Cyclical intermenstrual pain associated
                         with ovulation.

Features:
Common: up to 25% of women experience mid-cycle discomfort. Associated with ovaries (bilateral salpingo oophorectomy 'cures' it). Ranges from mild discomfort to severe pain.
Usually a non-cramping, non-radiating short-lasting pain, occuring only at mid-cycle which may or may not be associated with ovulation bleeding ('spotting').
May alternate from right to left side in different cycles (often helpful diagnostically).

HIRSUTISM

Definition:
Excess growth of hair in abnormal place on the body, i.e. non-female pattern hair on a female.

Pathophysiological mechanisms:
1. Physiological/racial, e.g. Southern European and Asian women.
2. Increased circulating androgens.
3. Increased end organ response.

Causes:
1. Physiological — racial and familial variation, pregnancy and post-menopausally.
2. Iatrogenic — drugs, e.g. phenytoin, steroids, antigonadotrophins.
3. Genetic abnormalities, e.g. intersex.
4. Endocrine disorders:
   adrenal/ovarian:
   - polycystic ovarian syndrome
   - adrenal hyperplasia
   - masculinising ovarian tumours
   - adrenal cortex tumours
   - Cushing's syndrome

   Others, e.g.
   - acromegaly

Virilism

This is a more generalised effect involving the development of male secondary sexual characteristics including:
  clitoral hypertrophy.
  breast atrophy.
  male pattern baldness.
  deeping of the voice.
  excessive body hair.

ACUTE VAGINAL BLEEDING

This is a common presenting symptom of gynaecological and obstetrical disorder in the Casualty Department. The condition may be life-threatening and urgent resuscitation with uncrossmatched blood may be required.

Causes:
1. Ectopic pregnancy.
2. Abortion — especially incomplete abortion.
3. Intra-uterine contraceptive device (usually recently fitted).
4. Heavy menstrual flow.
5. Ovulation — 'mid-cycle spotting'
6. Post-coital bleeding (q.v.).
7. Obstetric causes — show, abruption, placenta praevia.

Abnormal menstrual and non-menstrual genital bleeding

Abnormal menstrual and non-menstrual genital bleeding are frequent and important gynaecological symptoms, with a significance ranging from crippling heavy periods unassociated with serious underlying pathology, to the scant spotting which may be the only clue to an endometrial carcinoma. The main headings under which abnormal genital bleeding is considered are:

1. Abnormal menstrual bleeding
2. Non-menstrual bleeding: associated with pregnancy
   not associated with pregnancy.

Definitions:

Menarche:	age of onset of menstruation. Normal range in UK 10–16 years; average age 13½ years.
Menopause:	age at cessation of menstruation. Normal range in U.K. 45–60 years; average age 51 years (see p. 78).
Climacteric:	the period (as opposed to specific age) during which a woman changes from reproductive to non-reproductive ability.
Dysfunctional uterine bleeding:	abnormal uterine bleeding for which no organic cause can be found. The abnormality is assumed to be a disorder of the hypothalamic/pituitary/ovarian axis.

ABNORMAL MENSTRUAL BLEEDING

The terminology surrounding abnormal menstrual bleeding is confusing, many terms meaning different things to different people. For this reason the author prefers the use of plain English (thus D & C for menorrhagia' becomes less ambiguous as 'D & C

for heavy periods'). Nonetheless, the formal terms are
encountered and should be understood, and are therefore used
below.

In general terms it will be noted that abnormalities of flow are
usually due to local/genital causes, whilst abnormalities of cycle
timing are often due to systemic/endocrine causes.

N.B. Psycho-social problems may present as menstrual
abnormality.

Menorrhagia

Definition: cyclical menstrual bleeding which is
excessive in amount. No abnormality of
cycle is implied, but one may of course
be present.

Features: presents with excessive use of
towels/tampons; passing clots, flooding
and/or anaemia.

Causes:
1. Uterine polyps
2. Uterine fibroids *esp suberdometrial being extruded*
3. Endometrial hyperplasia (q.v.)
4. Pelvic inflammatory disease
5. Adenomyosis (*Fibromyomatous reaction to myometrial endometriosis*)
6. Endocrine disturbances
7. Systemic disease, e.g. liver disease
8. Dysfunctional uterine bleeding
9. Bleeding diathesis — should be excluded
   in the young teenager.

Cryptomenorrhoea (hypomenorrhoea)

Definition: cyclical menstrual bleeding of abnormally
small quantity (or spotting which may
occur at any time).
No abnormality of cycle is implied, but
one may of course be present.

Features: minimal menstrual loss, which may only
amount to a smear on the underwear.

Causes:
1. Endocrine disorders, e.g.
   hyperthyroidism
2. Scarring and obliteration of the
   endometrial cavity: (Asherman's
   syndrome)
3. General debility, e.g. tuberculosis
4. 'Physiological', i.e. as a normal variant
5. Oral contraceptive use

Polymenorrhoea

Definition: abnormally frequent (<21 days) menstrual cycle. No abnormality of flow is implied, but one may of course be present.

Features   self-evident condition, usually associated with anovulatory cycles.

Causes: ① Corpus luteum insufficiency
② Ovulatory failure
③ Disturbance of the hypothalamic/pituitary/ovarian axis.

Oligomenorrhoea

Definition: infrequent menstruation occuring at intervals in-between 6 weeks and 6 months. The causes are those of amenorrhoea (q.v.).

Amenorrhoea

Definition: absence of menstruation for 6 months or more. See p. 76.

Metrorrhagia

Definition: irregular vaginal bleeding occuring inbetween apparently normal periods. Synonymous with intermenstrual bleeding (q.v.).

Metropathia haemorrhagica

Definition: excessive menses at long intervals associated histologically with cystic endometrial hyperplasia, usually associated with anovulatory cycles.

MANAGEMENT OF ABNORMAL MENSTRUAL BLEEDING

Adequate history and examination (general and pelvic).

Investigations: full blood count (for anaemia)
biochemistry (e.g. LFT's)
21-day progesterone (if infertility is an associated problem)   As clinically indicated
endocrine investigation (e.g. thyroid function tests)

D & C: opinions vary concerning the timing (and indeed the necessity in some patients) of this procedure. A standard plan would be:

(1) Age 20 or less and adequate responses to hormone treatment (q.v.) — D & C not necessary.

(2) Age 20–40 and no suspicion of organic disease — D & C required, but may be deferred.

(3) Age over 40–D & C essential.

Other procedures, e.g. laparoscopy, may be needed in obscure cases in which there is suspicion of organic disease.

Treatment: the underlying disease is treated where appropriate. The remainder of patients will be said to have 'dysfunctional uterine bleeding' (q.v.): for these patients the treatment must be tailored to the severity of the bleeding and the individual patient's needs. Available options include:

General measures, e.g. correcting anaemia   *For 2-3 ⊕ only at first*

D & C in itself may be therapeutic   *2nd ½ ⊕*

Hormone treatment, e.g. OCP, progestogens, danazol   *General & horm. secretion*
(treatment of choice in younger patients)

Epsi-amino caproic acid   *— Stablises fibrin by inhibiting plasminogen*

Hysterectomy

The management of abnormal menstrual bleeding is summarised in the flow chart on page 32.

ENDOMETRIAL HYPERPLASIA

Incidence increases in the last menstrual decade.
Two types exist, differentiated histologically. Both cause abnormal uterine bleeding:

(1) Cystic hyperplasia

Benign
Caused by unopposed oestrogen stimulation.
Often associated with the clinical picture called 'metropathia haemorrhagica' (q.v.).
Histologically recognised by 'swiss cheese' appearance (large dilated endometrial glands) *but also GENERAL HYPERPLASIA*
Responds to progesterone treatment.

(2) Adenomatous (atypical) hyperplasia

20% risk of progression to invasive carcinoma.
Dependent on but not caused by oestrogen.
Histologically only endometrial glands are involved (c.f. cystic hyperplasia in which there is a more general hyperplasia).
Treatment (usually hysterectomy) is mandatory.

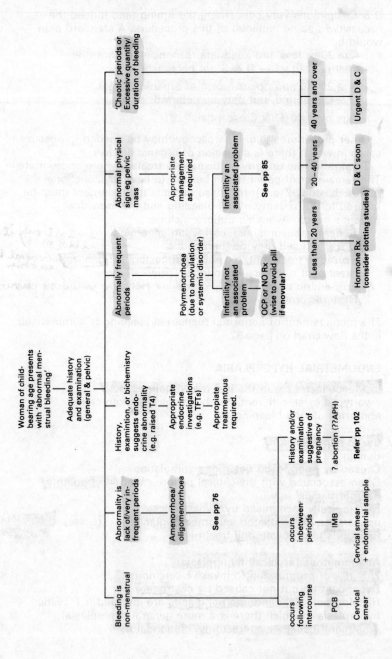

Fig. 14 Abnormal menstrual bleeding

NON-MENSTRUAL BLEEDING

Definition:
Any vaginal bleeding not associated with menstruation.

Unlike disordered menstrual bleeding, an identifiable pathological cause can usually be found.

Classification:
Intermenstrual bleeding: bleeding in between menstrual cycles.

Post-coital bleeding: bleeding after sexual intercourse.

Post-menopausal bleeding: bleeding after cessation of menstruation.

Bleeding in pregnancy (q.v.).

Common and/or important causes
Usefully considered anatomically. Those marked * are especially common.

Vulva and vagina:
Carcinoma
Inflammations
Urethral caruncle

Cervix:
'Erosions'
Polyp*
Carcinoma and dysplasia/carcinoma in-situ   *CIN II, III*

Uterine body:
Abortion*
IUCD*
Polyps
Hyperplasia
Carcinoma
Breakthrough bleeding (from OCP) and 'spotting' at time of ovulation.

Ovaries and Fallopian tubes:
Fallopian tube carcinoma
Oestrogen secreting ovarian tumours.

Management: Because of the risk of carcinoma in non-menstrual bleeding, urgent investigation and appropriate treatment is mandatory in all cases.

Gynaecological infections and inflammations

Inflammation, (including that due to infection), is a common gynaecological problem, and any part of the genital tract may be involved:

Vulvitis, including abscess of Bartholin's gland
Vaginitis, including abscess of Skene's gland
Cervicitis
Endometritis and pyometra
Salpingitis
Oöphoritis
Venereal diseases

Pelvic inflammatory disease is a general term for acute or chronic infection of the tubes and ovaries, often with involvement of the adjacent tissues.

VULVITIS

Inflammation of the vulva may be acute or chronic.

Aetiology

Infections:	Fungal infections, especially in the elderly, diabetics and after antibiotic therapy.
	Trichomonas vaginalis
	Venereal diseases
	Warts
	Herpes genitalis
Infestations:	Pediculosis pubis
	Threadworms
Mechanical/chemical:	Trauma
	Poor hygeine
	Urinary and faecal contamination
	Allergy to perfumes, soap, talc, Dettol etc

Miscellaneous:	Atrophic and dystrophic conditions
	Carcinoma
	Skin disorders — eczema, psoriasis, contact dermatitis, etc

Signs and Symptoms

Acute:	Pruritus
	Burning
	Erythema
	Oedema
	Bleeding
	Pain — may be very severe leading to an inability to walk or sit, and acute retention of urine
	Ulceration and/or vesicles
Chronic:	Less severe inflammation with minimal oedema
	Severe pruritus → excoriation → secondary infection
	Area involved may include
	mons
	perineum
	anus
	anal canal
	adjacent thighs
	Ulcerative lesions may be due to
	granuloma
	carcinoma
	melanoma
	End result may be destruction of the vulva

Diagnosis

History
General physical examination
Cervical and vulvar cytology
Local, endocervical, vaginal and urethral swabs
Full blood count
Urinalysis
Appropriate test for venereal disease if suspected

Treatment

General treatments:	Sitz baths
	Good local hygeine
	Avoid soaps
	perfumes

talcs
sprays
bath-oils
nylon underwear, tights and
trousers
Dry area thoroughly with hair-dryer after
washing
Oral antihistamines (which also cause
sedation which may reduce excoriation),
but avoid local antihistamines and local
anaesthetics which can themselves cause
sensitivity reactions
Topical steroids (*only* after treating local
infective causes)
Treating local irritation and cause will
reduce trauma/excoriation

Specific treatments: Education of elderly patients who may
well apply Dettol to the vulva to treat an
'infection' which commonly results in a
chemical vulvitis
Lice: gamma-benzene hexa-chloride
Scabies: benzoyl benzoate
Threadworms cause pruritis mainly at
night.
Eradicate with piperazine citrate
Canidiasis: treat diabetes mellitus if
present
Topical antifungals
Topical antifungals + steroid
Treat vaginal fungi
Trichomonas vaginalis: metronidazole
400 mg three times a day for 10 days.
Avoid intercourse for 2 weeks.
(It is only necessary to treat a woman's
consort if intercourse is not avoided for
this length of time.)

Warts: Local treatment with podophyllin
silver nitrate
cautery (diathermy)
excision
freezing
laser
Treat the partner.

VENEREAL DISEASES

Syphilis
Gonorrhoea
Chancroid
Non-specific urethritis
Herpes genitalis
Lymphogranuloma venereum
Granuloma inguinale
Trichomonas vaginalis

Syphilis

Syphilis is a contagious disease caused by the spirochaete
Treponema pallidum. It may be congenital (i.e. contracted in
utero), or acquired; the former may result in abortion, fetal death,
or congenital abnormality. In adults and children the disease may
be active and florid, or latent. Any tissue of the body may be
affected.

Stages

Primary (very infectious):	3–6 weeks after infection through an abrasion, a chancre forms. Spirochaetes can be obtained and identified under dark-ground illumination. Rarely observed in women. Often on the cervix but also on the vulva, lip, finger, anus. Almost painless Rubbery, painless glands Spontaneous healing with slight scar
Secondary (moderately infectious):	2 months after chancre Varied dermatological lesions which can mimic any lesion. Often a coppery coloured, maculo-papular rash. *Snail track ulcers* 80% have muco-cutaneous lesion 50% have generalised lymphadenopathy Alopecia Condyloma lata Rash heals with no scar, but may leave depigmentation or hyperpigmentation.
Tertiary (rarely infectious):	Appears within 3–10 years Gumma, due to endarteritis, of skin bone viscera

	Cardiovascular syphilis: aortitis aneurysms

Periostitis

Neurosyphilis: Tabes dorsalis
Charcot's joints
General paralysis of the insane *GPI*

Diagnosis: Positive Romberg's sign
Absent joint position sensation } neurosyphilis
Argyll-Robertson pupils

Serology: VDRL (screening test; +ve after 5–6 weeks, but don't forget yaws)
FTA-ABS (most sensitive; +ve 3–4 weeks)
RPCFT
TPHA   *WR ?*
TPI

Dark ground illumination

6x10⁵

Treatment: Penicillin 600,000 u/day i.m. daily for 10 days *or* 2.4 million u i.m. stat
Contact tracing
(Erythromycin 500 mg four times a day for 15 days in those allergic to penicillin).

Gonorrhoea

Gonorrhoea is a common infection caused by Neisseria gonorrhoeae, a Gram-negative, kidney-shaped, paired, usually intracellular organism. Symptoms usually appear 1–3 weeks after infection although up to 60% of women may be asymptomatic. Trichomonas vaginalis infection in the same patient is common. The adult vaginal epithelium is resistant to the organism which therefore colonises the

cervix
urethra
Skene's gland
Bartholin's gland
anus

Subsequent ascending infection to the endometrium, tubes and ovaries is common, with the formation of tubovarian abscesses.

Clinical manifestations of infection:

Dysuria
Discharge
Abscess:

      urethral
      cervical
      Skene's gland
      Bartholin's gland
      Tubo-ovarian

Vulvitis
Vaginitis (in children)
Dissemination via
  blood-stream causing

      iritis
      arthritis
      endo-carditis

Diagnosis:
      Gram-stained smear
      Culture (difficult)
      GCFT (becomes positive after 6 weeks)
      Reliable serology not available

Treatment:
      Penicillin (if not resistant) 4.8 mega-units [4.8×10^5]
        i.m. after probenecid 1 g orally $\frac{1}{2}$ hour
        before. (To block renal excretion)
      N.B. *Always* obtain blood for syphilis
        serology before starting treatment.

OR   Ampicillin 3.5 g orally after probenecid

OR   Tetracycline 1.5 g stat orally, then 0.5 g
        few times a day for 4 days.

One week after treatment check that the patient is not infectious. Check again at 2 weeks. Retreat as required.

Chancroid
Chancroid is an acute, contagious, localised lesion, consisting of small, painful, shallow irregular ulcers, associated with suppurating inguinal lymph nodes. It is caused by the short, slender, Gram-negative bacillus, *Haemophilus ducreyi.*

Diagnosis: Clinical findings

Treatment: Sulphonamides (Sulphadimidine 4 g
        daily for 10–14 days)
      Aspirate bubos (do not incise)
      Review patient for 3 months

Non-specific urethritis (NSU)
The development of more accurate diagnostic techniques has
increased the recognition of non-specific genital infection.

Organisms: Chlamydia trachomatis
                        Mycoplasma hominis — T strains

Features: Usually no symptoms, but may cause:
                           vaginal discharge
                           mild dysuria
                           frequency
                           pelvic pain
                           dyspareunia
                           Reiter's syndrome

Symptomatic in males who may develop Reiter's syndrome, a
serious complication, features of which are:
                           conjunctivitis
                           uveitis
                           polyarthritis

Diagnosis: By excluding gonorrhoea
                                     trichomonas
                                     candidiasis
                                     other causes of discharge

Treatment: Always treat the female partner of an
                           affected male.
                        Oxytetracycline 1 g daily for 2–3 weeks
                        Erythromycin stearate 1 g daily for 2–3
                           weeks
                        No intercourse or alcohol
                        20% relapse rate

Herpes genitalis
Herpes genitalis is the commonest cause of ulceration of the
vulva and cervix. It is caused by Herpes hominis virus type 2, and
is moderately contagious, developing 4–7 days after intercourse.
Relapses occur due to the carrier state.

Features: Itching and soreness before vesicles
                        Secondary infection can occur
                        Acute retention of urine requires
                           catheterisation
                    ?   Sacral radiculitis may occur
                        Clinical diagnosis confirmed by virus
                           culture

Treatment:	Symptomatic
	Idoxuridine
	Betadine skin paint
	Acyclovar
	No known cure

Lymphogranuloma venereum
This is a contagious infection caused by a Chlamydial organism.

Features:	Transient primary lesion
	Suppurative lymphangitis
	Serious local complications: oedema
	ulcer
	fistula

| *Diagnosis:* | Frei intra-dermal test |

Treatment:	Tetracycline 500 mg 6 hourly orally for
	14 days
	Aspirate bubos
	Follow-up patient for 6 months

Granuloma inguinale
This is a chronic granulomatous condition of the genitals which is rare in temperate climates, caused by a Gram-negative rod-shaped bacillus, Donovania granulomatis.

Features:	No lymphadenopathy
	Granulomatous mass
	Slow healing and scarring

| *Diagnosis:* | Donovan bodies |

| *Treatment:* | Streptomycin or tetracyclines |

Trichomonas vaginalis
Trichomonas vaginalis, a flagellate *protozoan* 15–30 μm long, with four flagellae and a membrane, is a common cause of infection in young women (up to 20%).

Clinical features:	Vaginitis
	Urethritis
	Cystitis
	Copious green/yellow offensive frothy
	discharge
	Irritation
	Soreness
	Dyspareunia

	Dysuria
	Symptom-free carriers
	Frequently associated with gonorrhoea
Diagnosis:	Direct microscopy
	Culture
	Papanicolou smear
Treatment:	Metronidazole 400 mg three times a day for 10 days
	Avoid intercourse for 14 days (see above)

Bartholinitis
Inflammation of Bartholin's gland.

Organisms:	Staphylococci
	Streptococci
	E. coli
	Gonococcus (rare)

An abscess may develope from an infected cyst

Treatment:	Incise
	Drain
	Marsupialise
	Culture pus for antibiotic sensitivity

Marsupialisation, in which the lining of the cavity is sutured to the skin, is a procedure more suited to cysts than abscesses, because in the latter the abscess wall is friable and the tissues oedematous.

Genital warts (syn. Condylomata acuminata)
Genital warts are caused by a papilloma virus with an incubation period of 1–6 months. The infection is acquired venereally.

Diagnosis:	Identified by appearance (but must be differentiated from the flat-topped Condyloma lata of syphilis)
	Biopsy (to exclude carcinoma-in-situ and frank carcinoma)
Treatment:	Podophyllin (not in pregnancy)
	Silver nitrate
	Cautery
	Excision
	Laser

VAGINITIS AND VAGINAL DISCHARGE

Vaginitis and vaginal discharge can be considered as occurring during three stages of life:

(1) **Pre-menarchal**

Causes:
Poor hygeine
Foreign body (organic or inorganic)
Threadworms
Sexual interference
Sarcoma botryoides (rare cause of blood-stained discharge)

Treatment:
Treat infecting agent
Remove foreign body (usually during examination under anaesthesia)
Local or oral oestrogens are occasionally indicated

(2) **Reproductive period**

Heavy "normal" discharge (usually increased at mid-cycle, due to ovulation, and pre-menstrually). Being pregnant and being on the 'pill' also cause heavy normal discharge.

Specific causes
Trichomonas vaginalis
Venereal diseases
Streptococci
Anaerobic organisms
Chlamydia
Retained tampon
Candidiasis (see below)
Non-specific

Candida albicans (Monilia)

This is a fungus infection, susceptibility to which is increased by oral contraceptives, antibiotics and diabetes mellitus.

Features:
Intense irritation and soreness
May spread to the thighs
Thick cheesey discharge
Red inflamed vaginal wall

Diagnosis:
Direct microscopy or Gram-staining (Test urine for sugar)

Treatment:
Anti-fungal pessaries and cream
Treat partner if required
Nystatin
Clotrimazole
Miconazole

Oral nystatin eliminates bowel reservoir of fungus

Non-specific
Sensitivity to contraceptive rubber
Sensitivity to spermicidal creams/foams
Inappropriate chemicals for douching

Peri/post-menopausal
In the peri- and post-menopausal period, atrophic vaginitis (due to low oestrogen levels) is very common. No specific organism is involved. The patient may complain of prolapse even though none is present.

Features: Purulent often blood-stained discharge (N.B. always exclude intra-uterine pathology whenever PMB presents)
Soreness

Treatment: Local or systemic oestrogens (after excluding malignancy) may be given

Abscess of Skene's gland
Gland opens at urethral margin
Develops a cyst or abscess

Differential diagnosis: Urethral diverticulum
Cyst of Gartner's duct (no urethral connection)
Urethrocoele (mid-line deformity)

CERVICITIS
Inflammation of the cervix which may be acute or chronic. May spread to uterus and parametrium.

Features: Purulent offensive discharge
May be associated with vulvo-vaginitis
Red oedematous cervix
Tender cervix/cervical excitation
Positive laboratory studies for aerobic and anaerobic pathogens

Causes: Acute cervicitis — gonococcus
puerperal infection
D+C
Chronic cervicitis — the sequel of acute cervicitis

Treatment: Antibiotics
                            Treat any cervical erosion

CERVICAL EROSION

Although called an erosion because of its raw appearance, this cervical lesion is not caused by erosion of the ectocervical squamous epithelium, but by a down-growth of the endo-cervical columnar epithelium onto the ecto-cervix.

Causes: Physiological — pregnancy
                                                menarche
                            Iatrogenic — combined 'pill'
                                                'mini-pill'

Features: Seldom occurs after the menopause
                            May resolve spontaneously (squamous
                                metaplasia → squamous epithelium)

CIN N.B. Cervical intra-epithelial neoplasia/dysplasia occurs in the
        transition zone between columnar and squamous
        epithelium.

Symptoms: Discharge
                            Intermenstrual bleeding
                            Post-coital bleeding
                            Often asymptomatic

Treatment (if   Take a cervical smear before:
symptomatic):   Cautery
                                Cryocautery
                                Laser

ENDOMETRITIS

This is infection of the endometrium which may occur:
        Post-abortion
        Post-partum
        Post-curretage
        Post-IUCD insertion
        Post-menopause (atrophic endometritis)

and as a result of: Ascending gonococcal infection
                            Descending tuberculous infection

Features: Pyrexia
                            Tachycardia
                            Uterine tenderness
                            Foul lochia
                            Pelvic peritonitis

Treatment: ERPC   Drainage — cervical dilatation
                                  Evacuate products of conception if
                                      present
                                  Antibiotics as appropriate
                                  Rest
                                  (Oestrogens in atrophic cases)
                                  Supportive therapy
                                  Exclude cervical or uterine carcinoma,
                                      especially with pyometra

Salpingitis

Salpingitis is a venereal infection of sexually active women which
is commonest in their late teens and early twenties.
IUCDs increase the risk, and are therefore not recommended for
contraception in young nulliparous women.

Causative organisms: Neisseria gonorrhoea
                         Chlamydia
                         TB (uncommon)

Pathology: Ascending vaginal infection
                                  ↓
                         Endocervical glands involved
                                  ↓
                         Superficial endometritis
                                  ↓
                         Endosalpingitis (bilateral)
                                  ↓
                         Exudate, adhesions, tubal occlusion
                                  ↓
                         Tubal abscess
                                  ↓
                         Pelvic peritonitis + oöphoritis
                         Tubo-ovarian abscess
                         Pyosalpinx
                         Hydrosalpinx
                                  ↓
                         Infertility

Features: Pain
                         Pyrexia
                         Tenderness + cervical excitation
                         Malaise
                         Dyspareunia
                         Vaginal discharge
                         Urethral discharge + or — frequency
                                                      Dysuria
                         Dysmenorrhoea
                         Menstrual disorders

Investigations:	Swabs — urethral endocervical high vaginal rectal MSU Blood cultures if required
Treatment:	Antibiotics once specimens taken — a penicillin metronidazole erythromycin or tetracycline for chlamydia

Remember to treat the sexual partners if indicated.

OÖPHORITIS/OVARIAN ABSCESS

This is uncommon as a primary condition, the tubes are usually also involved, (salpingo-oöphoritis or tubo-ovarian abscess).

Requires distinction from:	Ovarian tumour Endometriosis Intestinal and urinary tract disorder

ENDOMETRIOSIS

This is a condition in which the endometrium is found outside the uterine cavity. It is commonly found in the ovaries, Pouch of Douglas, vagina or umbilicus, and in scars after gynaecological operations. Bizarre presentations (e.g. cyclical haemoptysis) have been known to occur. Endometriosis within the myometrium is called adenomyosis.

Aetiology:	? retrograde menstruation leading to implantation ? implantation of fragments at operation ? Changes in peritoneal mesothelial cells to endometrial cells
Features:	Common in Europe and USA Rare in Negroes Common in nulliparous women Pelvic pain Dysmenorrhoea Menorrhagia Frequent periods Dyspareunia

Danazol — Anti-gonadotrophic agent.

- Infertility
- Pelvic pressure symptoms
  Uterine retroversion
  Thickening of the utero-sacral ligaments
- Nodules in the Pouch of Douglas
- Ovarian enlargement and tenderness
- (Chocolate cysts)

Diagnosis:
- History
- Examination
- Laparoscopy   with confirmatory
- Laporotomy   histopathology

Treatment:
Medical — continuous progestogen (e.g. norethisterone)
continuous danazol (an anti-gonadotrophic agent)
Surgical — diathermy of endometriomata (can be done down a laparoscope)
excision of endometriomata
TAH + BSO

Ponstan 500mg tds ≡ Mefanamic acid

Neoplasia and related disorders

Neoplasia may be congenital or acquired, benign or malignant, solid or cystic.

CONGENITAL

Vulva	Teratoma
	Haemangioma
Vagina	'Adenosis' (mothers given oestrogens)
	Cysts of Gartner's duct
Cervix	Mesonephric cysts (Wolffian duct remnant)
	Sarcoma botryoides
Uterus	Nil
Fallopian tubes	Fimbrial cysts
Ovaries	Parovarian cysts
	Hydatid of Morgagni
	Wolffian remnants

ACQUIRED (BENIGN OR MALIGNANT)

Vulva
The following list covers 'tumours' in the wildest possible sense, including lesions which cause enlargement of the vulva.

Benign:

Oedema
Haematoma
Bartholin's cyst/abscess
Sebaceous cyst
Lipoma
Granuloma
Haemangioma (senile; c.f. congenital)
Lymphangioma

Hidradenomas
Condylomata accuminata
Syphilis

Urethral prolapse / caruncle (cherry red)

Fibroma
Neurofibroma
Seborrhoeic keratosis

Management:
Excision if necessary.

Malignant (carcinoma of the vulva):
A rare condition.
4% of all primary genital cancers;
85–90% are squamous carcinomas
Others are undifferentiated
Occurs in post-menopausal women
Long history of pruritis and
blood-stained discharge
Association with vulvar dystrophies
Early lesions resemble
infection/inflammation
Late lesions ulcerated or polypoid
Commonly on anterior part of labia
majora
Biopsy essential

Unusual cancers:
Tumours of Bartholin's gland
Malignant melanoma
Rodent ulcer
Carcinoma of urethra

Management:
Biopsy
Result benign — continued observation
Result dysplastic — may be observed
with repeat biopsy.
Simply vulvectomy.
Result malignant — radical vulvectomy ±
radiotherapy to remaining groin and
pelvic nodes.

VULVAR DYSTROPHIES

The term vulvar dystrophy includes atrophic and hypertrophic
lesions, which produce circumscribed or widespread white skin.
In atrophic conditions the skin is white because there are few
blood vessels, in hypertrophy the whiteness occurs because the
thickened epidermis filters out the normal pink colour.
An inflammatory infiltrate is present.
Dysplasia and cancer can develop in both types of lesion.
Suspicious areas must be biopsied.
Evaluate lesions colposcopically if possible.

Treatment:	Atrophic lesions: topical testosterone ointment
	Hypertrophic lesions: topical steroids
	Topical oestrogens most useful for pre-menarchal patient. Both lesions symptomatically improved with vaseline.
	Steroids aggravate atrophic lesions.
	Simple vulvectomy occasionally required for chronic pruritis.
	Regular review necessary.

CARCINOMA OF THE VAGINA

Very rare, 1–2% of genital tract cancers

Present with —	Painless bleeding
	Pain
	Swelling
	An ulcerated or polypoid tumour
	Cachexia (late)

Types (primary):	Squamous (the majority)
	Adenocarcinoma (clear cell)
	Melanoma ⎫ Rare
	Sarcoma ⎭

Secondaries from:	Uterus
	Cervix
	Ovary
	Bladder
	Urethra
	Rectum
	Bowel
	Vulva
	Choriocarcinoma

Treatment:
This is difficult due to the proximity of the rectum and bladder. Mainstay is radiotherapy. *or topical cytotoxic therapy (5 fluorouracil*

Surgery:	Vaginectomy
	Pelvic exenteration

NB Vaginal cancers spreading to other genital structures are considered to be tumours of that structure.

To diagnose vaginal cancer the lesion must be clearly confined to the vagina.

CERVICAL NEOPLASIA

Benign 'tumours' of the cervix:

Nabothian cysts (blocked mucous glands)
Mesonephric cysts (Wolffian duct remnants)
Polyps (cause abnormal bleeding; remove)
Papillomas (95% benign; excise or cauterise)
Fibroids (uncommon)
Endometrioma (unusual; rarely large; excise or cauterise)

Carcinoma-in-situ
Cervical intra-epithelial neoplasia are graded 1, 2, and 3.
CIN 1 = mild dysplasia/abnormality
CIN 2 = moderate dysplasia
CIN 3 = severe dysplasia + CIS (carcinoma in situ)

Pathologists feel that whereas severe dysplasia is reversible, CIS is not. Cervical dysplasia is considered to be a pre-malignant condition. It is often asymptomatic, but may present 'classically' with post-coital bleeding, and also inter-menstrual bleeding and discharge. Detected by cervical cytology.

Treatment
This is by local ablation:

cone biopsy
radical cautery
cryocautery
laser
hysterectomy (abdominal or vaginal)

Carcinoma of the Cervix
This is a very interesting condition which is associated with intercourse, human papilloma virus infection, early age of first intercourse, multiparity, promiscuity, non-barrier methods of contraception and low socio-economic groups.
It causes 2000–2500 deaths per annum in England and Wales.

The previously held theory of a low incidence of this condition in the partners of circumcised males is no longer valid.

Associations with the pill probably reflect usage by young women starting intercourse as teenagers, with multiple partners, in social classes 4 and 5.

| Cell types: | Squamous carcinoma | 95% |
| | Adenocarcinoma | 5% |

Features

Early lesions (micro-invasive and occult) may be asymptomatic, detected by smear, colposcopy or biopsy.

Biopsy is essential. A micro-invasive or invasive cancer may lie below epithelium with CIN3/CIS.

Symptoms:	Post-coital bleeding
	Intermenstrual bleeding
	Post-menopausal bleeding
	Offensive blood-stained vaginal discharge
	Pelvic discomfort and pain
	Cachexia

Symptoms due to involvement of adjacent organs:	tenesmus and diarrhoea
	fistula
	haematuria
	renal failure (ureters)
	abdominal distension and vomiting (small bowel)
	referred nerve pain

Management:	History
	Examination
	Examination under anaesthesia with wedge or cone biopsy
	CXR IVU Lymphangiogram after confirmation of diagnosis
	MSU
	FBC + ESR
	U+E Creatinine clearance
	LFTs
	Pelvic ultrasound scan
	Bone scan in poorly differentiated lesions

Staging

The purpose of the above investigations is to stage the tumour, i.e. to assess how advanced it is and to detect metastases.

Treatment varies according to the stage.
The aim should be to give the maximum appropriate treatment with the minimum of side-effects/complications.

Figo staging

Stage 1	Confined to the cervix; la microinvasive; 1b others
Stage 2	Beyond cervix but not reaching pelvic side walls. Involving upper 2/3rds vagina.
Stage 3	Cancer extends to pelvic side wall or to lower 1/3rd vagina or there is hydronephrosis or a non-functioning kidney.
Stage 4	Cancer extends beyond pelvis. Involves bladder or rectal mucosa. Distant metastases.

Surgery and radiotherapy are each attended by morbidity and mortality, and combined treatment produces greater morbidity/mortality.
   Hence the need to stage accurately this disease in order to administer the single most appropriate therapy.

Treatment:

Stage 1	1a Microinvasive lesions 2 mm or less may be treated by cone biopsy or simple hysterectomy 1b Wertheim's hysterectomy or radiotherapy. Surgery better for young women. Results the same.
Stage 2	Radiotherapy + or − chemotherapy
Stage 3	Radiotherapy + or − chemotherapy
Stage 4	Radiotherapy + chemotherapy. Symptomatic and palliative treatment.

Chemotherapy useful in poorly differentiated tumours.
Survival

Stage 1	85%	
Stage 2	55%	5 year
Stage 3	30%	
Stage 4	10%	

Overall 5-year survival rate 50%.
  Regular follow-up is mandatory, ideally in a joint
gynaecology/radiotherapy clinic.

CARCINOMA OF THE ENDOMETRIUM

Used to be much less common than cervical cancer, but now
more common. Approximately 3% of women will develop the
disease if they live beyond 50 years.
Mean age 60–70 years.
Aetiology unknown.

Associated factors: Obesity
                       Diabetes mellitus
                       Hypertension
                       Low parity/nulliparity
                       Unopposed continuous oestrogen
                           therapy

Features: Post-menopausal bleeding
                       Abnormal peri-menopausal bleeding
                       Vaginal discharge
                       Uterus normal size or slightly large
                       Soft uterus
                       Associated factors noted above
                       Malignant endometrial cells in
                           vaginal/cervical smears and uterine
                           curettings

Definitive histological diagnosis made on uterine curettings which
are usually pale, friable and necrotic looking at curettage.

Pathology   Almost always adenocarcinoma
                       Occasionally squamous elements
                       Well differentiated tumours have a better
                           prognosis than poorly differentiated
                           lesions and those with squamous
                           elements.

Staging

Stage 1   Confined to uterus

Stage 2   Cancer extends to cervix

Stage 3   Cancer is outside the uterus but still in
                                 the pelvis

Stage 4   Spread into bladder or rectum or distant
                                 metastases

Management

Surgery   Total abdominal hysterectomy +
                                 bilateral salpingo-oophorectomy + cuff
                                 of vagina

Radiotherapy to vault by means of ovoids
   External radiotherapy depends on site of lesion and degree of
      penetration of myometrium. (Fundal lesions may spread to the
      nodes draining the ovaries.)
   Some surgeons prefer pre-operative radiotherapy
Progestogen therapy
NB Endometrial hyperplasia (cystic glandular) and adenomatous
   (microglandular) hyperplasia may both become cancer.

FIBROIDS

Leiomyoma (smooth muscle tumours) contain fibrous tissue as
   well and have a psuedo-capsule.
They are very common and influenced by oestrogen.
Caucasian women often present over the age of 30.
Large fibroids can occur at a much younger age in negros.

Pathology   Multiple
                                 Capsule of compressed myometrium
                                 Subserous +/− pedicle
                                 Intramural
                                 Submucous +/− pedicle
                                 Cervical
                                 Produce irregular uterine enlargement
                                 Degenerate

Types of   Atrophy (post-menopausal)
degeneration   Hyaline (most large fibroids)
(favourite examiners   Cystic (in hyaline areas)
question):   Calcification (post-menopausal large
                                    fibroids)
                                 Red (infarction, especially in pregnancy)
                                 Fatty
                                 Sarcomatous (malignant change; rare)

Pedunculated fibroids can undergo torsion.

Symptoms: Often none
                    Heavy periods
                    Painful periods
                    Frequent periods
                    Lower abdominal swelling
                    Pelvic pain/discomfort
                    May be associated with infertility
                    Pressure symptoms — stress
                                        incontinence
                                        urge incontinence
                                        frequency
                                        rectal pressure

                    Varicose veins ⎫
                    Piles   ⎬ Symptoms of
                    Ankle oedema   ⎭ venous obstruction

Fibroids can impact in the pelvis causing acute retention of urine.

Signs: Enlarged irregular uterus
                    Smooth swellings
                    Generally non-tender

Diagnostic aids: EUA + D+C
                    Ultra-sound scan
                    X-ray shows calcified fibroids

Treatment: Nil (if asymptomatic)
                    Hysterectomy
                    Myomectomy

Fibroids in   May cause — Pain (red degeneration)
pregnancy: Abnormal lie
                                Malpresentation
                                Obstruct labour
                                Uterine inertia
                                Post-partum haemorrhage

Never remove fibroids in pregnancy or at Caesarean section.
There may be fatal haemorrhage.

TROPHOBLASTIC DISEASE

This condition is 10 times more common in the Far East than in
Europe. Remember that normal trophoblast is invasive.
There are benign and malignant forms of the disease.

Hydatidiform mole

Diagnostic features:

Rapid uterine enlargement
Large for dates uterus
Excessive nausea and vomiting
Early onset of PET
Absent fetal heart
Snow storm appearance on ultra-sound scan
Uterine discomfort due to stretching
Grape-like vesicles passed
High urine HCG titres
Bilateral ovarian cysts (theca lutein) in half the cases

Distinguish from:

Multiple pregnancy
Hydramnios
Fibroids

Pathology/Aetiology
Cystic degeneration of chorionic villi
Occurs during first 18 weeks of pregnancy
Cause unknown
May cause —

Haemorrhage
Infection
Uterine rupture

Up to 20% of cases become malignant becoming choriocarcinoma

Treatment
Empty uterus —

Suction evacuation
Uterine stimulation (syntocinon; ↑ likelihood of prostaglandins) } embolisation
Hysterectomy
Hysterotomy (rare these days)

Curettage 7–10 days later
Careful follow-up
Patient avoids pregnancy (Pill) Pill delays tumour regression

Regular

CXR
Urinary HCG levels
β sub-unit HCG levels (serum)

Residual/persistent disease is treated with chemotherapy.

Choriocarcinoma
Curable
Early identification and treatment essential
Chemotherapy = Methotrexate (folic acid antagonist)
Metastasise to: Lungs
              Liver
              Brain
              Vagina
              Kidney
Best treated at specialist referral centre.

OVARIAN TUMOURS

Ovarian tumours may be benign or malignant, primary or
secondary, solid or cystic; most benign tumours have cystic
elements. Remember the congenital cysts at the start of the
chapter.

Benign

Cysts are usually physiological	Graafian follicle Corpus luteum
or retention cysts	Follicular cyst (from atretic follicles)
Endometriosis causes	chocolate cysts
Other benign tumours	Mucinous cystadenoma (can be massive) Serous cystadenoma Dermoid cyst Fibroma (can cause hydrothorax — Meig's syndrome)
Symptoms	May be none Pain with tortion, rupture or bleeding (may mimic ectopic pregnancy) Swelling Pressure effects Urinary retention Acute abdomen (through rupture)
Signs	Pelvic swelling Smooth Often mobile Dull to percussion Cystic on ultra-sound

Treatment	Generally any cyst >5 cm diameter should be removed if it does not go spontaneously. Smaller cyst should be kept under review.
	In pregnancy ovarian cysts are best removed at about 16 weeks gestation.
	Interest is being shown in the development of ultrasound screening of the ovaries for the early detection of ovarian cancer.

OVARIAN CARCINOMA

Ovarian carcinoma kills >3000 women in England and Wales per year, and about 2% of women in their 50s and 60s will die of the disease. Most patients present with advanced Stage 3 disease, and late presentation is common. Ovarian cancer is primary or secondary, solid or cystic.

Aetiology:	Unknown
	Malignant change in a benign lesion.
	Possibly more common in single women

Primary tumour types:	Mucinous cystadenocarcinoma
	Serous cystadenocarcinoma
	Endometrioid
	Granulosa cell
	Dysgerminoma

Secondary tumours from	Breast
	Stomach
	Colon (by direct and lymphatic spread)

Krukenberg tumours are secondary gastrointestinal tumours.

Staging

Stage 1	Confined to ovaries
	1a One ovary, no ascites
	1b Two ovaries, no ascites
	1c One or two ovaries with ascites
Stage 2	One or two ovaries with extension to the pelvis
Stage 3	Widespread intra-peritoneal metastases (Omentum commonly involved)
Stage 4	Distant metastases

Features	Late onset of symptoms
	Adnexal swelling
	Abdominal swelling/distension (tumour +/– ascites)
	Pressure symptoms (see Fibroids)
	Pain
	Cachexia
	Bowel symptoms
	May be associated with a second primary (often bowel)
	Often referred from physicians or general surgeons, having presented with non-gynaecological symptoms.
Investigations	FBC
	U+E
	LFTs
	Creatinine
	MSU
	CXR
	IVU
	Barium enema
Treatment	Surgical 'debulking' for all stages if possible
	'Debulk' = Total abdominal hysterectomy + Bilateral salpingo-oophorectomy + Omentectomy + Any other tumour greater than 2 cm diameter
	Adjuvant therapy — Radiotherapy for Stage 1b and 1c Chemotherapy for Stage 2,3 and 4, +/– radiotherapy to the abdomen
	Regular follow-up, with second look procedures at intervals, is essential.
	There must be a willingness to debulk further tumour at these reviews.

BASIC MANAGEMENT OF TERMINAL GYNAECOLOGICAL CANCER

Terminal care for the gynaecological cancer patient is the same as that for any cancer patient, but cancer of the female genital tract is often complicated by fistula, whether due to the disease process or as a complication of radiotherapy.

An account of terminal care should include the following points:

  Terminal admissions average 2 weeks
  (Teaching hospitals admit 2% of UK deaths)
  Pain relief without sedation
  Avoid constipation
  Control vomiting and nausea
  Companionship
  Occupy the mind
  Psychological support
  Good all-round communication
  Stop chemotherapy?
  Arrange residential care as required

Retroversion, genital prolapse and gynaecological urology

RETROVERSION OF THE UTERUS

Uterine retroversion should not be considered to be invariably pathological. It is a variant of the normal uterine position, and it is often asymptomatic.

Retroversion: the axis of the body of the uterus is
                             directed to the hollow of the sacrum.
                             The cervix points anteriorly.

Retroflexion: the axis of the body of the uterus is
                             directed to the hollow of the sacrum
                             BUT the axis of the cervix remains in the
                             normal axis.

Causes

Congenital   Adhesions ←—— Pelvic infection | Fixed

Acquired   ←—— Endometriosis | Retroversion

              Fibroids
              Occurs *during* uterine prolapse

Features   May be none
                             Dyspareunia
                             Subfertility
                             Incarceration of gravid uterus with acute
                                 urinary retention
                             Incarceration of gravid uterus with
                                 abortion

Management   Treat cause
                             Correct position with an Hodge pessary
                             Ventrosuspension/shortening of the
                                 round ligaments

Caution: Any pelvic surgery can cause adhesions
                                  and tubal damage with subsequent
                                  infertility.

Incarceration of the gravid uterus requires catheterisation of the
patient, and may require anteversion of the uterus under general
anaesthesia.

GENITAL PROLAPSE

The walls of the vagina, vaginal fornices and uterus can prolapse.
A protrusion such as an enterocoele can be considered as a true
hernia.

Types   Cystocoele
                                  Urethrocoele
                                  Rectocoele
                                  Enterocoele
                                  Uterine prolapse (vault descent)

Definitions

Cystocoele: Prolapse of the posterior bladder wall
                                  and trigone and anterior vaginal wall.
                                  Usually occurs with an urethrocoele

Urethrocoele: Prolapse of the urethra, usually with the
                                  bladder neck

Rectocoele: Prolapse of the anterior rectal wall with
                                  the posterior vaginal wall. A recto-
                                  vaginal hernia

Enterocoele: Hernia of the Pouch of Douglas through
                                  the posterior vaginal fornix, containing
                                  small bowel

Uterine prolapse: An abnormal descent of the uterus
                                  through the vagina

Aetiology

All prolapse share a common aetiology: weakness of stuctures
supporting the pelvic organs.

Supporting   Pelvic floor (levator ani + perineal body)
structures: Ligaments + connective tissue of pelvic
                                      fascia
                                  Cardinal ligaments
                                  Uterosacral ligaments
                                  Pubo-cervical fascia

Weakening factors:	Childbirth (? episiotomy protects)
	Post-menopausal atrophy
	Raised intra-abdominal pressure:
	Obesity
	Chronic cough
	Chronic constipation
	Abdominal hysterectomy

Features

Cystocoele and urethrocoele:	Vaginal fullness
	'Something falling out' SCD
	Incomplete bladder emptying
	Stress incontinence
	Need to push lump up to pass urine.
	Soft reducible mass in introitus
	Increased bulge with straining

Rectocoele:	Difficult defaecation
	Vaginal fullness
	'Something falling out'
	Soft reducible mass posterior vaginal wall
	Thin perineum — skin, no muscle

Enterocoele:	Vaginal discomfort
	'Something falling down'
	Bulging mass posterior fornix
	Associated with uterine prolapse/post TAH
	Post-menopausal women
	Simultaneous rectal and vaginal examination distinguishes from rectocoele

Uterine prolapse:	Firm mass lower vagina
	Cervix through introitus
	Inside-out vagina
	Vaginal fullness
	'Something coming down'
	Sacral back-ache
	Ulceration causing post-menopausal bleeding
	1° descent in vagina
	2° descent to introitus
	3° descent outside vagina; no spontaneous reduction

Remember: Genital prolapse is best examined with Sim's speculum.

Management   History
                        General examination
                        Gynaecological examination and cervical
                          smear

Treatment
Conservative or surgical.

Conservative: None if asymptomatic
                       Vaginal pessary (permanent or
                         temporary): Ring
                                      Shelf
                       Pelvic floor exercises

Surgery: Anterior repair
                       Posterior repair
                       Vaginal hysterectomy
                       Manchester repair

Pregnancy not contraindicated after a repair
Vaginal delivery probably unwise after a successful repair for
stress incontinence.

GYNAECOLOGICAL UROLOGY   See notes

Urinary incontinence
This is the involuntary loss of urine; intermittent or continuous.

Types: Enuresis
                     1 True incontinence
                       Stress incontinence
                       Urgency incontinence
                       Overflow incontinence

Enuresis
Definition: Uncontrolled emptying of bladder at
                         night.
                       Normal up to 3 years of age.   N < 3 −6
                       Investigate after 6 years for
                         physiological, anatomical or
                         psychological abnormality.

True incontinence
Congenital: Ectopic ureter
                       Ectopia vesicae

Acquired: Trauma to urethra/bladder neck
                          Senile dementia
                     MS   Disseminated sclerosis
                          Paraplegia
                          Fistula
                            (a) Uretero-vaginal
                            (b) Vesico-vaginal

Stress incontinence
Definition: The involuntary loss of urine with a
                              sudden rise in intra-abdominal pressure.
                          Common. About 50% of all women
                              >45 years.
                          Parous

Aetiology: Loss of support at urethro-vesical junction
                          Bladder base descent, resulting in a
                              shorter, wider urethra. Less resistance
                              to flow.

Causes: All causes of genital prolapse above.

Urgency incontinence
Definition: Urgent desire to void urine followed by
                              the involuntary loss of urine.
                          Can occur with stress incontinence.
                          Due to detrusor instability.

Causes: - Infection
                          - Atrophic changes
                          - Irradiation
                          - Calculi
                          Diverticula   ?
                    - MS DS
                          - Urethritis
                          - Neurogenic bladder

Overflow incontinence
                          Overdistension of the bladder resulting in
                              a dribbling incontinence.

Aetiology: Urethral stenosis
                          After vaginal surgery
                          Post-partum
                          Loss of bladder sensation
                              due to age or neurological
                              disorder.

Diagnosis of incontinence (see the flow-chart)
The history is the most important factor in making the correct diagnosis.
Examination
Special investigations

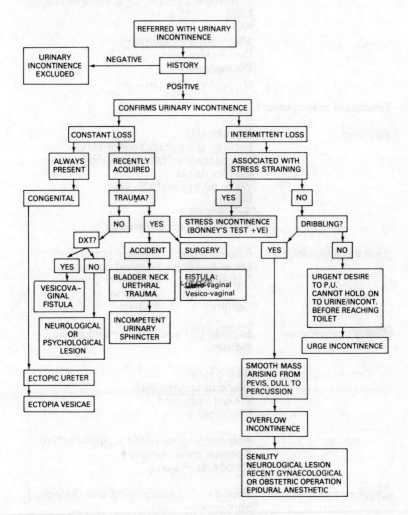

Fig. 15 Diagnosis of incontinence

Examination:	With a full bladder
	Sim's speculum
	? Bonney's test

Special tests:	? Pyridium instilled into bladder for fistula
	? Methylene blue i.v. for ureteric fistula
	MSU
	IVU
	Micturating cystogram
	Cystometry
	Cystoscopy
	Urinary dynamics

Treatment/management

Enuresis	Exclude UTI
	Exclude renal tract abnormality
	Empty bladder before retiring
	No late drinks
	Wake during night to void
	Alarms
	Imipramine
	Support + encouragement

True incontinence	Ectopic ureter	Surgical correction
	Ectopia vesicae	Surgical correction
	Fistula	Closure or urinary diversion
	Senility	Catheter

| Stress incontinence | Exclude UTI and urgency and pelvic masses |

Conservative:	Ring pessary
	Pelvic floor exercises
	Weight reduction
	Oestrogens

Surgical:	Anterior vaginal repair (colporrhaphy)
	Remove pelvic tumours
	Colposuspension

| Urgency incontinence | Exclude UTI, neurological and urological abnormality |

Surgery:	NEVER indicated
	Bladder drill
	Anti-cholinergic drugs *may* help

| *Overflow*
incontinence | Catheterise
Rest bladder
Correction of stenosis
Permanent catheter for neurological deficit |

Cystitis

Inflammation of the bladder (acute or chronic). Much more common in females than males.

| *Common causative*
organisms | *E. coli*
Enterobacter
Klebsiella
Strep. faecalis
Proteus
Psuedomonas
Don't forget TB |

| *Symptoms* | Dysuria (burning/painful micturition)
Urgency
Frequency
Pain — supra-pubic and and low back
Haematuria — occassionally gross
Fever |

| *Aetiology* | Bacterial infection: Poor hygiene
Sexual intercourse
Instrumentation
Radiation
Fistula — colo-vesical |

| *Investigation* | MSU — microscopy, culture and sensitivity.
Positive = >5 WBC/HPF or >10^5 organisms/HPF
Recurrent cystitis requires: IVU
Cystoscopy |

IVU and cystoscopy are mandatory when there has been haematuria.

| *Treatment* | Correct aetiological factor if possible
Education
Antibiotics
High fluid intake
Mist. Pot. Cit. or pyridium for dysuria
Post-coital antibiotic prophylaxis
Long term antibiotic prophylaxis |

Urethritis
Inflammation of the urethra, acute or chronic.

Common causative organism — Gonococcus
Non-gonococcal (non-   (1)Chlamydia trachomatis
specific) urethritis   (2)T-strain mycoplasma
                             Corynebacterium

Symptoms	Dysuria
	Frequency
	(Abscess may occasionally form)
Aetiology	Sexual intercourse
	Instrumentation
Investigation	Swabs — urethral + cervical
	(Special swabs and transport medium
	for chlamydia)
	Serological tests for syphilis
	MSU

Treatment
(1) VD suspected: Refer to special clinic
                        Rapid identification of organism
                        Contact tracing
                                            -48×10^5
(2) Gonorrhoea: A penicillin + probenecid 1–2 g orally
                        to block renal excretion of penicillin
                        Tetracycline for resistant strains

(3) NSU: Tetracycline/oxytetracycline
                        Avoid alcohol for 2 weeks

Haematuria
Blood in the urine. Colours urine red or brown depending on the
amount of blood and the urine pH. Slight haematuria may
produce no colour change, being detected by microscopy.

Haematuria
Painless: Renal
                        Vesical
                        Casts = glomerulonephritis
                        No casts, think of renal or bladder
                        tumour
                        Stones
                        Polycystic kidney

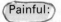 **Painful:**   Stone (renal colic)
                          Infection — Cystitis
                                  Pyelonephritis

Remember schistosomaiasis in immigrant patients.

Urethral stricture
Congenital or acquired

| Acquired | Trauma | Obstetric | peri-urethral |
| | | Coital | fibrosis |

Symptoms: Dysuria
                      Slow stream
                      Infection

Special Tests: Urethroscopy
                      Cysto-urethrography

Treatment: Urethral dilatation

Urethral Caruncle
Small, red, fleshy, sensitive 'growth' at posterior margin of the external urinary meatus.
Single.
Comprises vascular granulation tissue + thin stratified transitional or squamous epithelium.
May be infected. Probably caused by infection.

Symptoms: Bleeding: PMB or haematuria
                      Dysuria
                      Frequency
                      Pain
                      Urgency
                      Dyspareunia
                      Malignant change (very rare)

Treatment: Excision
                      Cautery
                      Oestrogen cream

Urethral mucosal prolapse
May be confused with caruncle. May be distinguished from caruncle because it surrounds the external urethral meatus.
It may be present in children.

Treatment: Excision

Urethral diverticulum
Usually found in the mid-portion of the urethra, and the patient is usually over middle-age. They lie in the mid-line.

Cause:	Rupture of para-urethral (Wolffian) remnant
	Injury
Symptoms:	Para-urethral swelling
	Dysuria
	Purulent urethral discharge
	Dyspareunia
Distinguish between:	Urethrocoele — a mid-line swelling
	Abscess of Skene's gland — opens at urethral margin
	Cyst of Gartner's duct — no urethral connection

Urethral Carcinoma
Rare.
Squamous or transitional cell; occasionally adenocarcinoma

Symptoms:	Haematuria
	Local mass
Lymphatic drainage:	Lower urethra — Inguinal glands
	Upper urethra — Obturator glands and internal iliac glands
Treatment:	Radiotherapy
	Surgery

The prognosis is poor.

Pyelonephritis
A diffuse, often bilateral, pyogenic infection of the kidney.
Clinically infection of the renal pelvis cannot be distinguished from infection of the renal parenchyma.
Extremely serious for the pregnant patient.
Associated with pre-term labour and fetal mortality.

Aetiology:	Urinary stasis
	Bacterial invasion
	Infection
	E. coli in 85% of infections
	Catheterisation
	Haematogenous spread (most common with Staphylococcal bacteraemia)
Symptoms:	Fever
	Rigor
	Pain/tenderness in renal angle
	Dysuria
	Haematuria
	Frequency
	Urgency
	Nausea + vomiting
Investigations:	MSU = Pyuria
	Organisms >100,000/ml on culture
	FBC + ESR
	IVU if haematuria
	Cystoscopy
Treatment:	Fluids — oral/i.v.
	Antibiotics (after MSU)
	MSU at regular intervals
	In pregnancy — long-term antibiotics

N.B. Recurrent infection is either a relapse (the same organism), or a re-infection (different organism).

Relapsing infections —	Renal scource
	May require parenteral antibiotic
Re-infection —	Bladder infections usually

Endocrine and related disorders

AMENORRHOEA

Definition: Absence of menstruation for 6 months or more.

The distinction between primary and secondary amenorrhoea is of little use clinically as the causes overlap (but note that secondary amenorrhoea implies that there has been an intact functioning genital tract). The term 'post-pill amenorrhoea' should also be avoided since not only is it uncertain whether the condition exists as a discrete entity, but also its use as a 'diagnosis' may divert attention from more serious causes.

Oligomenorrhoea is defined as menstruation occuring at intervals of greater than 6 weeks, up to 6 months. In practice it is not usefully considered as a separate entity, since the causes of oligomenorrhoea are in effect those of amenorrhoea.

Incidence: The incidence of amenorrhoea in women of reproductive years is approximately 1–2%.

Causes

Physiological: Pre-menarche and post-menopausally. Pregnancy and often during lactation.

Pathological:
i.e. occuring in the absence of pregnancy in a woman of child-bearing age (16 years the upper limit of normal for the menarche, to 40 years the lower limit for the menopause).

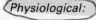

Anatomical (1% of all cases):
                                congenital, e.g. vaginal atresia.
                                aquired, e.g. endometrial fibrosis
                                (Asherman's syndrome)

(2) *Endocrine* (99% of all cases):

    (1) Primary endocrine organ failure (12%):
        primary hypothalamic failure
        primary pituitary failure
        primary ovarian failure

    (2) Hyperprolactinaemia (20%):
        pituitary tumours
        drug induced hyperprolactinaemia, e.g.
        phenothiazines
        hypothyroidism (causes raised TSH).

    (3) Polycystic ovarian syndrome

    (4) Misceallaneous (rare — ? 2% in all):
        thyroid disease
        diabetes mellitus

    (5) Hypothalamic disorders (60%):
        feed-back disorders (often with marked
        psychological element, e.g. anorexia
        nervosa)
        cycle initiation defect.

Investigations

History and clinical examination:

Especially for:
    Weight loss — psychiatric disorders
    Symptoms/signs suggestive of thyroid
      disease
    Drug history
    Hirsutism/virilism
    Genital tract abnormality (e.g.
      obstruction due to imporferate hymen).
    N.B. Cryptomenorrhoea is concealed
    menstruation due to an imperforate
    hymen.

Endocrine investigations:

    Serum prolactin (if raised, XR (or CT scan)
      sella turcica)
    Progesterone challenge test: if no
      withdrawal bleed, proceed to combined
      oestrogen and progesterone challenge.
    Serum FSH/LH assay
    Free thyroxine index (if indicated).
    Clomiphene response if infertility an
      associated problem.

These investigations, and how they are used to arrive at a diagnosis, are summarised in the flow chart (Fig. 16).

Added to these, chromosome studies for the karyotype may be useful.

Day Progesterone should be 30-60 Nmol/l.

Management

Depends on: the cause of the amenorrhoea
                         whether infertility is an associated
                         problem

If infertility is not an associated problem, contraception will
usually be required in addition to the treatment outlined below in
the table.

Treatment of amenorrhoea

Diagnosis	Treatment — Infertility is a problem	Infertility not a problem
Primary hypothalamic/pituitary failure	Gonadotrophins (beware over stimulation).	Oestrogen replacement therapy if symptoms require
Primary ovarian failure	Pregnancy impossible	Oestrogen replacement for symptomatic deficiency
Hyperprolactinaemia	No difference in treatment: Drug induced — stop drug Primary hypothyroidism — thyroxine Tumours — small — bromocriptine — large — (especially if pregnant) pituitary ablation as tumour may grow rapidly. Visual fields must be checked regularly	
Polycystic ovarian syndrome	Clomiphene (Wedge resection of ovary)	Tumour — excise Hirsutism — OCP ($\uparrow$ SHBG) or cyproterone acetate and oestrogen
'Hypothalamic disorders'	Clomiphene Gonadotrophins Psychiatric referral	Anorexia nervosa and related dsorders

Sex hormon binding globu

MENOPAUSE

By definition, the last menstrual period.
    Average in UK — 51 years.
    Preceded by the climacteric, which also continues after the true
menopause (i.e. the last menstrual period).
    The primary event of the menopause (and climacteric) is
ovarian failure resulting in decreased oestrogen production: it is
this decrease in oestrogen which results in the physiological and
symptomatic effects of the menopause.

Physiological consequences of the menopause:	Amenorrhoea
	Vulval and vaginal atrophy
	Thinning of the endometrium
	Body of the uterus shrinks relative to the cervix
	Increased osteoporosis
	Breast atrophy
	Urinary tract atrophy

Symptoms:	Hot flushes
	Atrophic vulvo-vaginitis
	Urinary disturbances
	Psychiatric disturbances
	Increased incidence of ischaemic heart disease
	Increased incidence of fractures

Clinically useful symptoms suggestive of the climacteric:
Any of the above may indicate the presence of the climateric, but in particular:

Hot flushes and sweats
Lengthening menstrual cycles
Mood and sleep disturbances

Post-menopausal hormone pattern:	FSH greatly increased (can be used diagnostically)
	LH moderately raised
	Oestrogen levels fall
	Prolactin levels fall
	Progesterone levels fall

Possible treatment(s) for menopausal symptoms (treatment is not always indicated):

Oestrogens:	Only hot flushes and vulvo-vaginitis are known to respond
	Osteoporosis may be prevented (but not reversed)
	Oestrogen therapy is not without risk: therapy should be cyclical and be combined with 12 days progestogen/progesterone to reduce risk of endometrial carcinoma
	Therapy is contraindicated in many conditions (including oestrogen dependent tumours, hypertension and acute liver disease)
	For these reasons oestrogens should only be used to treat symptoms

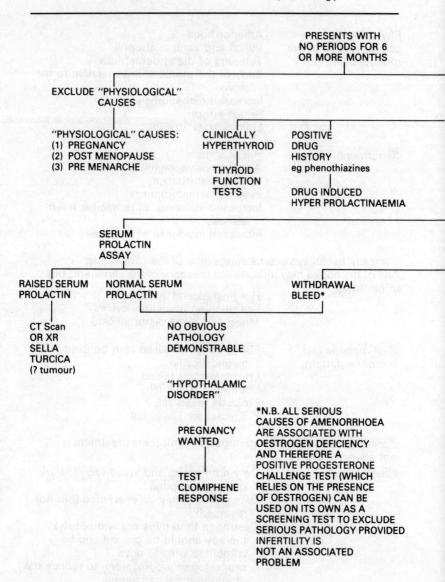

Fig. 16 Investigation of amenorrhoea

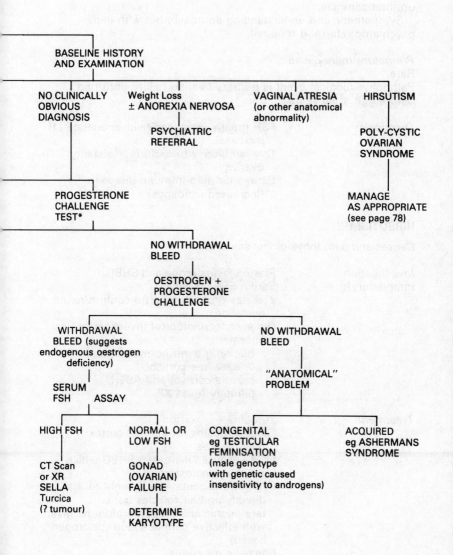

BASELINE HISTORY
AND EXAMINATION

NO CLINICALLY
OBVIOUS
DIAGNOSIS

Weight Loss
± ANOREXIA NERVOSA

PSYCHIATRIC
REFERRAL

VAGINAL ATRESIA
(or other anatomical
abnormality)

HIRSUTISM

POLY-CYSTIC
OVARIAN
SYNDROME

PROGESTERONE
CHALLENGE
TEST*

MANAGE
AS APPROPRIATE
(see page 78)

NO WITHDRAWAL
BLEED

OESTROGEN +
PROGESTERONE
CHALLENGE

WITHDRAWAL
BLEED (suggests
endogenous oestrogen
deficiency)

NO WITHDRAWAL
BLEED

"ANATOMICAL"
PROBLEM

SERUM
FSH   ASSAY

HIGH FSH

NORMAL OR
LOW FSH

CONGENITAL
eg TESTICULAR
FEMINISATION
(male genotype
with genetic caused
insensitivity to androgens)

ACQUIRED
eg ASHERMANS
SYNDROME

CT Scan
or XR
SELLA
Turcica
(? tumour)

GONAD
(OVARIAN)
FAILURE

DETERMINE
KARYOTYPE

Surgery (rare) e.g. dilation of the lower urethra; excision of urethral caruncle.

Sympathetic and understanding approach, but with early psychiatric referral if required.

Premature menopause
Rare.
Pathophysiological event is primary ovarian failure occurring before age of 40 years.

Diagnosis:	FSH greatly increased (with moderate LH increase)
	Ovarian biopsy to exclude 'resistant ovaries'.
	Screen for auto-immune disease (increased incidence)

HIRSUTISM

Causes and pathophysiology: see p. 26.

Investigation (mandatory):	Plasma testosterone and SHBG.
	Serum FSH/LH assay.
	21st day progesterone (to confirm/refute ovulation)
	Other endocrinological investigations as indicated:
	human growth hormone assay
	urinary free cortisol
	plasma cortisol and ACTH
	pituitary fossa XR
Treatment:	Tumours — excision
	Glucocorticoids for adrenal cortex disturbances
	OCP — causes increased SHBG which mops up testosterone
	Cyproterone acetate — thought to act directly on hair follicles but is teratogenic and must therefore be given with effective contraception (oestrogen based)
	Cosmetic measures

CHILDHOOD GYNAECOLOGY

Gynaecological problems are rare in childhood. The following list provides an indication of the type of problems encountered:

Congenital abnormalities of the genital tract.

Intersex states (abnormal sexual differentiation):
gonads female pseudohermaphroditism (female gonads; apparently external genitalia)
gonads male pseudohermaphroditism (male gonads; apparently female external genitalia)
true hermaphroditism (very rare)

Vulvo-vaginitis and discharge (usually due to foreign body) and other genital infections (including sexually transmitted diseases)

Trauma to the genital tract

Precocious puberty

Delayed sexual maturation

Tumours, e.g. sarcoma botryoides

PREMENSTRUAL TENSION SYNDROME

Consists of a symptom complex appearing 1–10 days before the onset of menstruation. Represents an exageration of the normal premenstrual phase and is only defined as the premenstrual tension syndrome if it is sufficiently severe to disturb the patients life. It usually appears when the patient is in her 30s and it has shown to be an important cause of increased suicide and violent crime amongst women in the premenstrual phase.

Symptoms:

1. Psychological disturbance:
   irritability
   moodiness and weepiness
   feeling of tension
   depression

2. Fluid retention:
   bloated abdomen
   tense tender breasts
   'sausage fingers'

3. Miscellaneous:
   headaches and migraines
   faints
   backache
   easy bruising

Treatment: Suppression of ovulation (with which it
                is associated) by use of the oral
                contraceptive pill
                Progesterone/progestogen therapy in
                2nd half of cycle
                Diuretics
                Avoid tranquillizers and anti-depressants
                — psychiatric referral should be
                arranged if indicated
                Mefanamic acid
                Supportive counselling

Infertility

Infertility and its investigation, management and treatment is easy to understand. In basic terms (which can provide the framework for an essay plan) there must be
— a sperm
— an ovum
— the opportunity for them to get together

Definitions and statistics

Infertility   is the failure to conceive after 12 to 18 months of regular intercourse without contraception. Subfertility is synonymous. Approximately 1 in 10 couples are affected.

It may be either *primary*, in which the woman has never conceived, or *secondary*, in which there is failure to conceive despite one or more successful or unsuccessful pregnancies in the past.

Sterility   means that there is no ability to conceive.

In about 35% of infertile couples, the male is at fault.
In about 30% of infertile couples, the female is at fault.
In the remainder, both are at fault.
In the presence of normal coital activity:
  42% of menstrual cycles result in no conception
  42% of menstrual cycles result in normal fertilised ova
  16% of menstrual cycles result in an ova which will abort
If a woman misses a period, there is approximately a 70% chance of a normal pregnancy, and a 30% chance of a miscarriage.

85

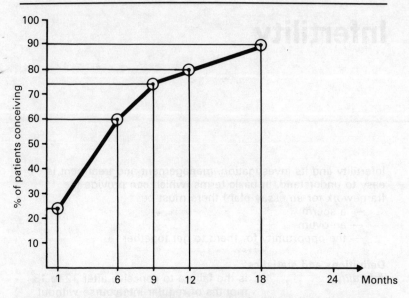

Fig. 17 The percentage of women who conceive after regular unprotected intercourse increases with time. Note that by 18 months 90% will have conceived

Thorough work-up will identify the cause in 90% of couples. Appropriate treatment will lead to pregnancy in about 40% of couples treated.

A proportion of 'infertile' women will conceive following the first consultation with no treatment once they have 'off-loaded' their problem onto the medical practitioner.

Causes

Female

General: Timing of intercourse
                            Frequency of intercourse
                            Activities after intercourse: getting up to
                                                          micturate or
                                                          douche

Anatomical:

① Congenital — Uterine absence
Uterine hypoplasia
Gonadal dysgenesis
② Acquired — (a) Tubal occlusion at any
portion of the tube by:
Gonorrhoea
Chlamydia
Tuberculosis
(b) Appendicitis and pelvic abscess
(c) Pelvic adhesions after surgery
Pelvic adhesions after ectopic pregnancy
(d) Abnormalities due to endometriosis
(e) Aschermann's syndrome
(f) Fibroids, especially submucous fibroids
which act like IUCDs
(g) Cervical and vaginal infections, by
making the local environment hostile
to sperms
(h) Iatrogenic: tubal ligation

Endocrine:

(a) Premature ovarian failure
(b) Pituitary failure
(c) Raised prolactin due to an adenoma or
micro-adenomata
(d) Thyroid disorder
(e) Adrenal disorder
(f) Polycystic ovary syndrome with raised
serum testosterone
(g) Obesity
(h) Anorexia nervosa (some authorities
believe that amenorrhoea occurs
below a weight of about 7 stone); recent
weight loss is important   *Wt at which you started menstruating*
(i) Diabetes mellitus

Male

Oligospermia means that there is a reduced number of sperms present in the ejaculate. Azoospermia means that there are no sperms present.

Causes of
oligospermia/
azoospermia:

Mumps orchitis
Diabetes mellitus
Alcohol
Smoking
Herniorrhaphy — especially in infancy
Operations for non-descent/maldescent
of the testis
Exposure to radiation

Chemotherapy
Drugs — salazopyrine; dapsone and
    many others
Toxic substances — lead; copper
Tight underpants
Varicocoele
Hydrocoele
Cryptorchids (remember that an ectopic
    testis can undergo malignant change)

Normal semen analysis suggests possible psychosexual
problems, e.g. impotence, premature ejaculation, inability to
ejaculate.

Retrograde ejaculation caused by:	Bladder neck surgery prostatectomy

Post-coital MSU in retrograde ejaculation contains sperms.

Normal semen analysis values:	Volume 2–6 ml
	Viscosity Full liquefaction in 60 mins
	Sperm density 40–250 × 10⁶/ml
	Motility 60%
	Vitality 35% dead
	Morphology 60% normal

Aphorism:	4 ml with more than 40 million/ml with 40% abnormal forms and 40% dead

Sperm counts less than 10^6 per ml or 25×10^6 per ejaculate are
uncommon in infertile males.
    3–5% of men show evidence of auto-immunity with circulating
antibodies to their own sperms.

Antibodies	auto-agglutinating auto-immobilising

Auto-agglutinating antibodies cause clumping of sperm on semen
analysis.
Auto-immobilising antibodies cause poor mobility on semen
analysis.

Auto-immunity may be caused by:	Obstruction to the vas deferens (and may therefore be present after reversal of male sterilisation) Inflammatory prostatitis Orchitis Testicular Biopsy

The presence of auto antibodies may reduce the pregnancy rate by 50% or more.

INVESTIGATION

Diagnosis = History + Examination + Special Tests

A scheme for the investigation of the infertile couple is described below using flow charts. As a useful exercise, the student might like to join the separate flow charts together to clarify how they inter-relate.

Ideally the couple are seen together.

More realistically, the woman is seen as near to mid-cycle as possible, having had intercourse within the previous 12 hours, this for the purpose of performing a post-coital test.

Points to highlight in the history:

1. Coital history
2. Acquired anatomical changes
3. Contraceptive history
4. Obstetric history
5. Drug ingestion
6. Alcohol consumption (male partner)
7. Menstrual history
8. Galactorrhoea (suggests raised prolactin)

On examination look especially for:

1. Thyroid enlargement/disorder
2. Galactorrhoea
3. Physique — hirsutes
4. Genitalia — abnormality
5. Cervical and vaginal inflammation and discharge (Take a smear if not done within the past 2 years)
6. Take bacteriological swabs if indicated
7. Assess stringiness of cervical mucous (Spinnbarkheit)
8. Aspirate from the endocervix for the post-coital test
9. On bimanual pelvic examination look for:
   a. Uterine abnormality
   b. Thickening of the tubes
   c. Adnexal masses
      Thickening of the utero-sacral ligaments
   d. Tenderness

Special Tests:

FBC ESR
VD Serology

Rubella titres (so that you don't have to
    worry about contacts if your treatment
    is successful)
21-day progesterone
Serum prolactin
Chest X-ray if none done within 2 years
    or immigrant
Consider thyroid function tests
If amenorrhoeic/oligomenorrhoeic do
    TFTs FSH + LH
Endometrial biopsy, specimens being
    sent for TB culture as well as
    histopathology. Such biopsies may be
    taken later at the time of laparoscopy,
    ideally in the pre-menstrual phase. The
    non-invasive investigations should be
    completed first.

By now we should be able to start sorting our infertile women
into different groups like this:

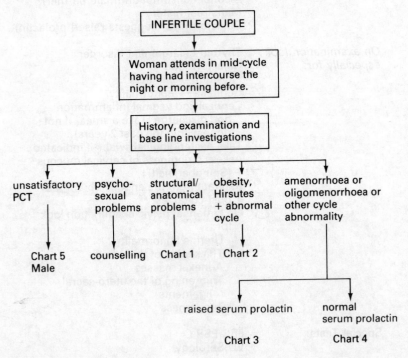

Fig. 18 Guide to flow charts

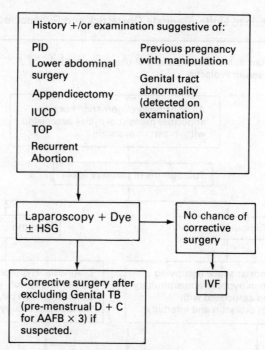

Fig. 19 Flow chart 1   Structural/anatomical problems

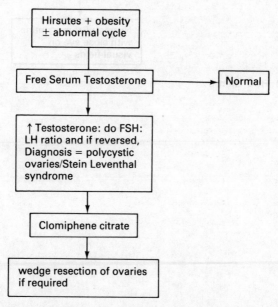

Fig. 20 Flow chart 2   Hirsutes + obesity + abnormal cycle

Flow Chart 3: Menstrual abnormalities associated
with ↑ serum Prolactin

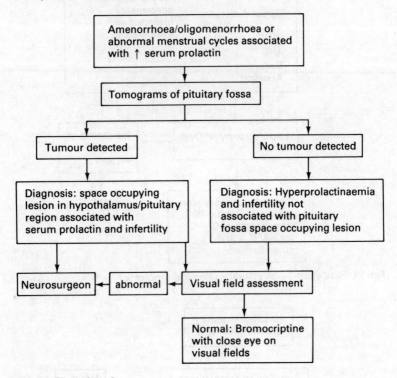

Fig. 21 Flow chart 3

Flow Chart 4 menstrual abnormality associated
with normal serum prolactin

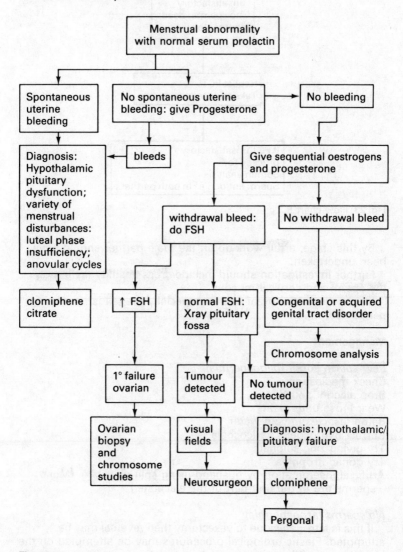

Fig. 22 Flow chart 4

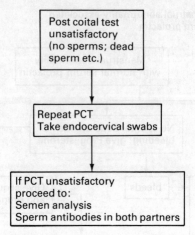

Fig. 23 Flow chart 5

By this stage, a full work-up on the male partner should have been undertaken.

Further investigation should include cross-hostility testing of the sperm and cervical mucous.

Electron microscopy of sperm, especially the tail is now being performed.

Management

Low sperm count (*oligospermia*)
Check medication
Stop alcohol abuse
Wear loose underpants
Bathe testicles in cold water
Correct hydrocoele, varicocoele
Try giving zinc sulphate
Try gonadotrophins
Artificial insemination by husband using split ejaculate. (Most sperms are in the first part of the ejaculate.)

No sperms (*azoospermia*)
If this is iatrogenic due to vasectomy then reversal may be attempted. Plastic urological procedures may be attempted on the bladder neck if there is retrograde ejaculation.

Artificial insemination by donor.

Finally, if there is no chance of the couple conceiving, they should be counselled about adoption and the several adoption agencies.

Contraception, sterilisation, abortion

Contraception
Traditional
Chemical
Mechanical
Hormonal
Intra-uterine contraceptive device (IUCD)
Sterilisation

Pearl Index
Measure of effectiveness of contraceptive.

$$PI = \frac{\text{Total Accidental Pregnancies}}{\text{Total Months of Contraceptive Exposure}} \times 1200$$

= Number of pregnancies/100 years of contraceptive exposure
i.e. the lower the PI, the better the contraceptive.

Traditional
Male:	Coitus interruptus	(PI = 10–38)
	Coitus saxonicus ?	
Female:	Lactation (prolongation of)	(PI = 24–26)
	Rhythm (safe period)	(PI = 24–38)

Chemical
Vaginal douche	(PI = 21–41)
Spermical foam, jelly, cream,	(PI = 4–43)
'C-film' (may also mechanically	
inhibit sperm and provide	
prophylaxis against STD)	

Side-effects:
Sensitisation to agents used (either partner)

Mechanical

Male:	Condom	(PI = 7–28)
	(May also provide	
	prophylaxis against	
	STD)	

Female:	Diaphragm (Dutch cap)	(PI = 4–35)
	Cervical caps	
	Both should be used with	
	spermicidal cream	

Hormonal

Oral contraceptive agents
Combined pill (high or low oestrogen)   (PI = 0.03–0.1)
Progestogen only (mini-pill)   (PI = 2–7)
The pill provides the most effective form of
contraception.

Mechanism of action
 (i) Oestrogen component inhibits ovulation by inhibiting FSH
     production by the anterior pituitary
 (ii) Inhibiting LH releasing factor production LHRH
 (iii) Progestogen component keeps cervical mucous viscid to the
     detriment of sperm transport, and produces hostile changes
     in the endometrium.
   Progestogen only pills are taken daily at the same time.

Contraindications to combined pill
Pregnancy
DVT and thrombo-embolic disorders
Liver disease and recurrent jaundice
Breast and uterine cancer
Sickle cell disease
Hyperlipidaemia

Be cautious about use in:
Diabetes mellitus
Hypertension
Patients over 35 years who smoke (progestogen only pill OK)
The obese
Lactating mothers → DVT + Smilk
? Epilepsy
Cardiac and renal disease

Side-effects
Oestrogen
Weight gain, fluid retention
Nausea, vomiting
Headache
Hypertension
Impairment of liver function
Benign hepatic tumours
Reduced venous flow in legs
Increase in size of fibroids

Progestogen
Breast tenderness
Acne
Depression
Headache
Hirsutism
Loss of libido
Weight gain (steady)
Dry vagina
Reduced menstrual loss
Cervical erosion

Drug interactions reducing the effect of oral contraceptives
Antibiotics
Barbiturates ·
Carbamazepine
Phenytoin
Rifampicin
(Gastrointestinal disturbance)

Oral contraceptives reduce the effect of:
Antihypertensive drugs
Diuretics
Warfarin
Phenindione
Tricyclic antidepressants
Oral hypoglycaemics
Insulin

Injectable contraceptives
Medroxyprogesterone acetate (a progestogen)
    (PI = 0.5–1.5)
Useful for short-term contraception
    (1) after vasectomy
    (2) rubella immunisation
Use may be followed by transient infertility and irregular cycles.
Now approved for long term contraception.

Intra-uterine contraceptive devices (IUCDs)
Pearl Index (overall for different types) 0.8–5.8
   New copper bearing devices (such as Novaguard) may be left
in for 4 years.

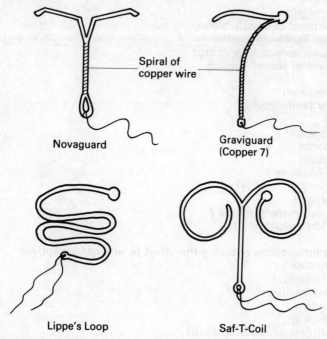

Spiral of
copper wire

Novaguard

Graviguard
(Copper 7)

Lippe's Loop

Saf-T-Coil

Fig. 24 Examples of currently used intra-uterine contraceptive devices
(coils)

Side-effects/complications
Excessive uterine bleeding
Pain
Expulsion: 10% during 1st year; mainly in first few
                           months after insertion
                           About 20% expulsions unnoticed and
                           followed by pregnancy

Perforation of uterus: about 1:1000 insertions

Device detected by
X-ray: AP and lateral of pelvis
                           AP and lateral of abdomen

Ultrasound scan may help.
Contrast in uterus may help (sound or dye)

| Pelvic inflammatory disease | <30 days probably due to IUCD
>30 days probably venereal in origin |

Coil may be left in for initial treatment.
1:20 chance of ectopic pregnancy if become pregnant with IUCD in situ.
If intra-uterine pregnancy plus coil, gentle attempt at removal with patient's informed consent.
If coil is stuck, leave in situ.
50% chance of abortion. No effect on fetus.

Sterilisation

Male:	Vasectomy
Female:	Tubal Occlusion
Pre-operative considerations:	Age (most women requesting reversal of sterilisation were sterilised below the age of 30) Marital stability Medical fitness Counselling Previous abdominal/pelvic surgery
Vasectomy	Safe Simple Usually done under local anaesthesia 1 cm segment of vas defereus removed Not immediately effective: absence of sperm must be confirmed in two ejaculates, one month apart.
Tubal Occlusion	
Many different methods:	laparoscopic laparotomy
Laparoscopic	Falope rings (tiny elastic bands) Clips Diathermy coagulation
Laparotomy	Fimbriectomy Salpingectomy Pomeroy tubal ligation Hysterectomy

Although each method is intended to be irreversible, permanence cannot be guaranteed, with the exception of salpingectomy and hysterectomy.

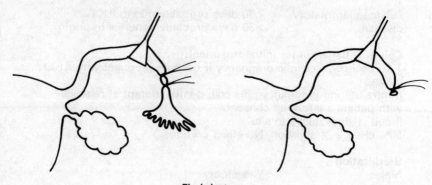

Fimbriectomy

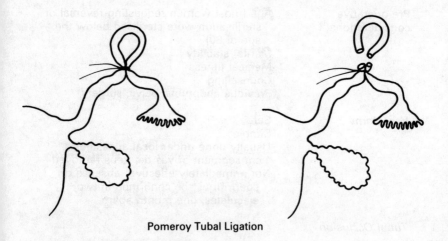

Pomeroy Tubal Ligation

Fig. 25 Two methods of female sterilisation

Complications
Hazards of any anaesthetic
Hazards of any operation
Diathermy coagulation: risk of thermal damage to other
  structures
Psychological/psychiatric sequelae

Side-effects
Approximately 20–40% of women subsequently undergo
  hysterectomy for menstrual problems.

Induced abortion
Considered for medical or non-medical reasons.

Medical reasons: Fetal abnormality
                      Blighted ovum/missed abortion
                      Renal disease
                      Certain cardiac disorders
                      Recurrent severe pre-eclampsia
                      Previous vesico-vaginal fistula repair
                      Pulmonary TB
                      Leukaemia
                      Psychiatric disorder

Abortions in United Kingdom legal under 1967 Abortion Act,
under four clauses:
  1. Risk to life of pregnant woman
  2. Risk of injury to physical or mental health of woman
  3. Risk of injury to physical or mental health of existing
     child(ren) of the woman's family
  4. Physical or mental fetal abnormality
Majority performed under clause 2.

Methods
Vacuum aspiration   1st trimester (occasionally up to 16
                       weeks gestation)

NB All vaginal suction terminations risk cervical damage and
    subsequent mid-trimester abortion.

Mid-trimester
Extra- or intra-amniotic prostaglandins
Intra-amniotic urea
Hysterotomy and hysterectomy (unusual in modern practice)

Complications of early pregnancy

ABORTION

Definition:

Termination of pregnancy (spontaneous or induced) before 28 weeks duration. It should be remembered that whilst the terms miscarriage and abortion are medically synonymous, for patients they are often not.

This definition is more legal than medical in that the time limit is set at 28 weeks, since this used to be considered the limit of fetal viability.

Recent experience has shown this not to be the case: Special Care Baby Units with intensive care facilities can now 'save' pre-term infants of 24 weeks, and it is getting lower still.

Incidence:

Very common: quoted rates vary between 1 in every 2 conceptions to 1 in every 10, the difficulty being in recognising the event. A useful day to day figure is 1 in 3.

Abortion is an extremely important subject, not least because it represents a major source of maternal morbidity and mortality.

Classification:

Spontaneous abortion (as opposed to induced abortion, see p. 101) may be viewed as a process which passes through identifiable stages. This progression provides a classification based on which stage has been reached:
Threatened
Inevitable
Incomplete
Complete
or
Missed.

Additional classification is by:	Time:
	  early 0–12 weeks
	  late (mid-trimester) 12–28 weeks

	Infection present or absent:
	  septic
	  non-septic

	Frequency of occurence:
	  isolated
	  habitual (recurrent)

Clinical features of abortion
Abortion may present at any of the stages listed above.

Threatened Abortion
Definition:

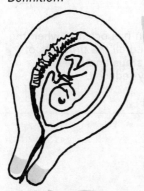

Fig. 26 Threatened abortion

Any uterine bleeding in a woman with an intra-uterine pregnancy of 28 weeks or less gestation occuring in the absence of cervical dilation, ± pain.

The extragenital features of pregnancy (delayed menstruation, breast tenderness, etc) are usually present.

The blood may be red or brown depending on the volume of blood lost and/or the time interval since the bleeding occurred.

Backache may be present but pain is usually not a feature: its presence suggests progression to the next stage — inevitable abortion.

Inevitable abortion
Definition:

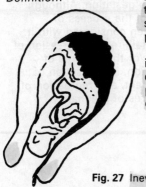

Inevitable abortion occurs when threatened abortion progresses to the stage of cervical dilation. Loss of the pregnancy is now 'inevitable'.

Progression from threatened to inevitable abortion is often indicated by cramping lower abdominal pain. (Sacral pain strongly suggests cervical dilatation.)

Bleeding is usually more profuse.

Fig. 27 Inevitable abortion

Incomplete abortion
Definition:

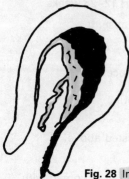

Incomplete abortion occurs when abortion progresses to the point when some but not all of the products of conception have been expelled from the uterus.

Pain ('cramps' as the uterus tries to expel the residual products) and bleeding (because the uterus is unable to contract adequately because the residual products) are usually present.

Fig. 28 Incomplete abortion

Complete abortion
Definition:

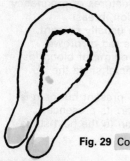

Complete abortion has occured when the uterus has expelled all the products of conception. Pain stops and bleeding stops or is greatly reduced.

Fig. 29 Complete abortion

Missed abortion
Definition:

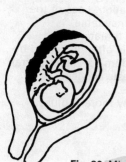

Fetal death in utero without its expulsion prior to 28 weeks gestation. Although not strictly part of the process of abortion, it is often considered with it.

Presents with failure of pregression of the pregnancy +/or the features of threatened abortion, i.e. cessation of uterine enlargement, and regression of the clinical features of pregnancy.

Fig. 30 Missed abortion

Missed Abortion
Diagnosis:

Negative pregnancy test following previously positive test. Ultrasound: no fetal heart movements; serial ultrasound scans: no fetal growth.

Management:

Opinions vary — either:
1. Non-intervention with subsequent spontaneous expulsion of the products of conception. Psychological support for the mother is important, or:
2. if diagnosis has been made for 4 or more weeks (or earlier if maternal psychiatric or medical complications indicate) induction of abortion, usually by prostaglandin or oxytocic administration (if uterus >12–14 weeks size) or surgical evacuation (if uterus <12–14 weeks size).

Complications:

Sepsis
Disseminated intravascular coagulation
Psychological disturbance of mother

Recurrent (Habitual) abortion
Definition:

Three or more consecutive abortions which may be early or mid-trimester. The implication is that the abortions are due to recurrent factors rather than accidental causes and therefore investigation and treatment where possible is appropriate.

Causes:

Any cause of abortion but in particular:
Parental chromosome abnormality
Maternal uterine abnormality
Chronic maternal ill health (e.g. diabetes, renal failure)
Incompetent cervix (usually causes mid-trimester abortion q.v.)
Maternal infection — CMV, rubella, toxoplasmosis, brucellosis.
In practice, a cause is often not found in recurrent 1st trimester abortion (c.f. mid-trimester abortion).

Investigation:	Chromosome analysis
	Hysterosalpingogram and cervicogram
	WR, CXR, urineanalysis (i.e. screening general health of the patient)
	Progesterone assay
	Rubella, CMV, toxoplasma, herpes, titres, (TORCH screen)

Treatment:	Apart from correction of specific identifiable causes, no treatment has been proven to prevent recurrent early abortion.
	The following have been tried:
	progesterone supplements (not those based on testosterone)
	specific attention to diet and vitamins (especially folic acid and vitamin C pre-conception)
	rest and correction of anaemia
	avoid intercourse at times of greatest risk

Mid-trimester (late) abortion

In contrast to 1st trimester abortion, mid-trimester abortion is less common, but more often recurrent when it does occur, and a cause is usually identifiable. Investigation after the first loss is therefore appropriate.

Causes:	Incompetent cervix (recognised by painless abortion — the fetus 'drops out' and often a history of previous gynaecological surgery involving cervical trauma is present)
	Maternal uterine abnormality
	Fetal abnormality and intra-uterine death (the expelled fetus should be sent for laboratory examination if possible)
	High order multiple pregnancy and/or hydramnios
	Maternal ill health

Treatment:	*Macdonald* Shirodkar (or similar) suture for incompetent cervix (now becoming controversial)
	Surgical correction of uterine abnormality
	Treatment of maternal ill health as appropriate

General causes of abortion

Patients (and examiners) often wish to know why abortion
occurs. Often in a particular case the cause is not known, but the
following provides a list of possible causes. Special
considerations apply to mid-trimester abortion (q.v.).

Fetal Causes (most — Gross malformation
common and not — Chromosome abnormality
recurrent): ③ — Failure of implantation

 in all

Maternal Causes: — Corpus luteum insufficiency
④ — Uterine abnormalities
— Cervical incompetence
— Maternal ill health/infection.

Mutual factors: ① — Failure of immune tolerance.

In day to day practice abortion without obvious cause is usually
assumed to be due to fetal abnormality. Some patients may
appreciate the idea that when there is fetal abnormality, abortion
represents nature's way of getting rid of 'bad' fetuses.

Management of abortion

Diagnosis: The history and general examination will
                        suggest the diagnosis.
                        Opinions vary concerning the
                        advisability of vaginal examination.
                        Usually gentle examination is acceptable
                        to the patient (and most consultants) and
                        allows differentiation between threatened
                        and inevitable abortion.
                        Ultrasound scan
                        Pregnancy test

Treatment: The treatment depends on the stage:

                        Threatened abortion: 1 in 3 will progress
                        to inevitable abortion and it is doubtful
                        whether any therapy alters the outcome;
                        however, any or all of the following may
                        be used:
                            Bed rest
                            Sedation, especially for active
                                patients for whom bed rest is difficult
                            Avoidance of intercourse
                            Progesterone supplements
                            Reassurance to the mother that if
                                the pregnancy does continue to fetus
                                is likely to be normal

Inevitable and incomplete abortion:
General measures including treatment of
shock and/or infection if present.
If required, urgent control of
haemorrhage may be attempted by
removal of products or with ergometrine
0.5 mg i.m./i.v.
The definitive treatment is surgical
evacuation of the uterus — ERPC
(evacuation of retained products of
conception).

Complete abortion:
Accurately diagnosed, requires no
treatment.
If in doubt, best to perform ERPC.
(Ultrasound scan is now being used to
exclude the presence of retained
products.)

ECTOPIC PREGNANCY

Definition:

Pregnancy in which implantation of the
fertilised ovum occurs outside the
uterine cavity.

Incidence:

0.3% of normal births (not pregnancies)
5–10% recurrence rate (in addition to
which a woman has only 1 in 3 chance
of a normal pregnancy after an ectopic
pregnancy).

Mortality:

Ectopic pregnancy accounts for 9% of
maternal mortality.

Risk factors:

Previous ectopic pregnancy
Pelvic inflammatory disease (especially
due to gonnococcus and tuberculosis)
Tubal surgery
Intra-uterine contraceptive device per se
(not as a result of infection caused by
the device) but note that this is a relative
increase only: the absolute rate is of
course decreased since the device is
itself a contraceptive.
Increased incidence in negroes
Progesterone only pills (see note about
relative and absolute rates above)

Sites of implantation:

Ampulla of tube } tubal pregnancy
Isthmus of tube } (95% of all ectopic pregnancies)

Ovary: rare
Abdomen: rare
Cervix: very rare

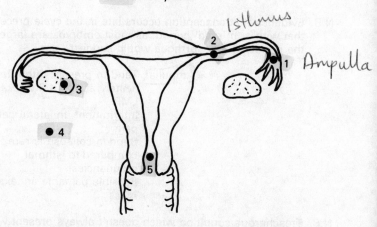

Isthmus

Ampulla

Fig. 31 Sites of implantation in ectopic pregnancy. (1) Ampulla of tube; (2) isthmus of tube; (3) ovary; (4) abdominal cavity; (5) cervix

Pathophysiology/
outcome:

Depends on site:
Isthmus of tube — tubal rupture
Ampulla of tube — tubal rupture or abortion (extrusion via end of tube)
Ovary — usually ruptures
Abdomen — may proceed to term

Clinical features:

Clinical features of early pregnancy: delayed menstruation, breast changes, early morning sickness, frequency of micturition
Postural hypotension
Further features depend on the site:
Isthmus: Tend to present 'acutely' at about 4 weeks from LMP. Severe lower abdominal ± shoulder tip (referred diaphragmatic) pain
Dark vaginal blood loss, typically after the pain
Shock and signs of peritonism
"Prune juice" vaginal loss

Vaginal tenderness with marked cervical excitation on vaginal examination (which should only be done in hospital because of the risk of provoking further bleeding)

N.B. Evidence that conception occurs late in the cycle preceeding that with a 'missed' period, as most embryos are larger than the period of amenorrhoea would suggest.

(Ampulla:) Tend to present rather less acutely at about 6 weeks from LMP
Intermittent unilateral pelvic pain
Sudden collapse is rare compared to isthmal pregnancies.
Possible palpable adnexal mass

N.B. Treacherous condition which doesn't always present with classical symptoms; can be 'chronic' as in the broad ligament.

Differential diagnosis: Only common diagnoses are listed:
Appendicitis
Pelvic inflammatory disease
Ruptured corpus luteum cyst/ovarian cyst
Uterine abortion
Urinary tract infection

Management of ectopic pregnancy
The management depends on the gravity of the situation.
Seriously ill shocked patient with 'certain' diagnosis:
Resuscitation = IVI with blood, continue and perform laparotomy as soon as possible. Usual definitive procedure: salpingectomy
Probable ectopic pregnancy, but patient not gravely ill:
Diagnostic EUA ± laparoscopy followed by laparotomy and salpingectomy if required
Patient in whom the diagnosis only a possibility:
Ultrasound scan of pelvis: note intra-uterine pregnancy does not exclude co-existent ectopic pregnancy: ectopic pregnancy must be specifically looked for.

Pregnancy test may be positive or negative and is therefore of little help.
Curettage of the uterus (for whatever reason) may produce intra-uterine decidua but no chorionic tissue, or the Arias Stella Phenomenon may be seen.
These two findings suggest the presence of an ectopic pregnancy.

N.B. Conservative surgery for ectopic becoming more common i.e., tube segment + ectopic resected only.

TROPHOBLAST DISEASE

Rare and somewhat conceptually bizarre but important spectrum of 'diseases' ranging from normal trophoblast tissue (which itself is capable of invasion and metastasis) to choriocarcinoma. The spectrum includes:

Normal 'metastatic' trophoblast (e,g, in the lungs)
Hydatidiform mole
Invasive mole
Choriocarcinoma

The matter is further confused by the fact that one manifestation of the disease may progress to or arise from another manifestation of the disease (see figure 32 below).
   A finer discussion of the disease is given on pp 58–60.

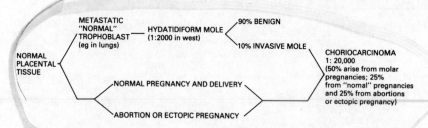

Fig. 32 Trophoblast disease: inter-relations and rates of incidence

OBSTETRICS

Antenatal care. 1: Normal

NORMAL PHYSIOLOGY

Physiological reference values are changed in pregnancy and therefore it is necessary to know the nature of these changes in order to be able to interpret values determined during pregnancy.

Endocrine changes during pregnancy
See also pp 16–18 which contains additional information on endocrinology.

Oestrogens (including oestradiol, oestriol)
Oestrogen levels rise progressively in maternal plasma during pregnancy, this rise being reflected in urinary oestrogen secretion (see figure 33).

Serial assay of oestriol (which is produced mainly by the fetus) can be used clinically to monitor fetal wellbeing, especially in late pregnancy (going out of fashion).

Progesterone
As its name suggests, represents the main pro-gestational hormone. Overall levels rise during pregnancy as shown in figure 34.

Human chorionic gonadotrophin (HCG)
Levels rise rapidly in early pregnancy both in maternal plasma and urine and as such provide a useful basis for a pregnancy test.

Levels plateau after 10–12 weeks and do not change much thereafter (see figure 35).

Human placental lactogen (HPL)
Produced by the placenta in progressively larger quantities as the pregnancy proceeds: (see figure 36).

May be used clinically as a placental function test (going out of use).

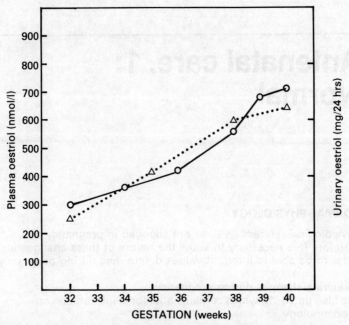

Fig. 33 Normal pregnancy. Maternal plasma (○) and urinary (△) oestriol concentration during the last trimester; the rise shown may be absent if there is fetal pathology

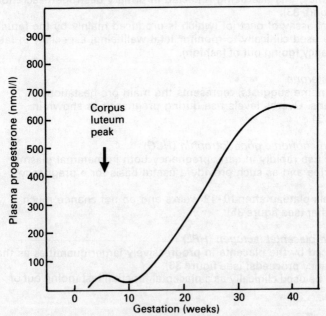

Fig. 34 Normal pregnancy: maternal plasma progesterone concentration

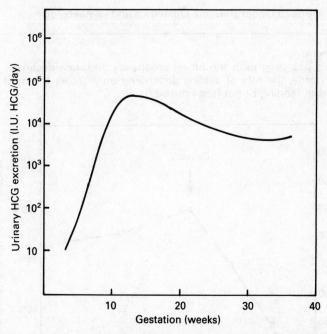

Fig. 35 Normal pregnancy: maternal urinary HCG excretion (note semi-log plot)

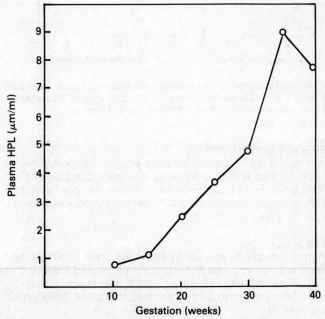

Fig. 36 Normal pregnancy: maternal plasma HPL concentration

Prolactin
Levels rise progressively during pregnancy and then decline afterwards, the rate of decline depending on whether the mother is breast feeding or not (see figure 37).

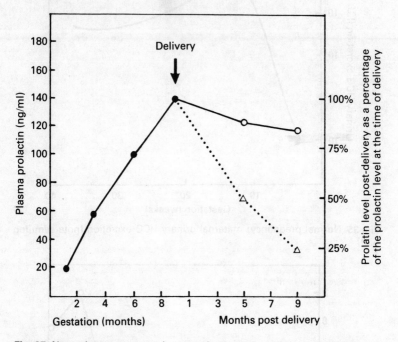

Fig. 37 Normal pregnancy and puerperium: maternal plasma prolactin levels before and after delivery showing effect of mainly breast feeding (solid line) and mainly not breast feeding (dotted line)

Insulin and glucose tolerance
Glucose tolerance is impaired during pregnancy (partly due to HPL) and for this reason pregnancy has been described as 'diabetogenic'. Figure 38 illustrates glucose tolerance in pregnant and non-pregnant women. The clinical consequences of these changes vary (see pp 149–151).

Thyroid status
Pregnancy induces a 'pseudohyperthyroid' state in which the pregnant woman appears hyperthyroid (increased BMR, increased total T4, increased cardiac output, etc) but in reality remains biochemically euthyroid in that her free thyroxine index and TSH remain normal.

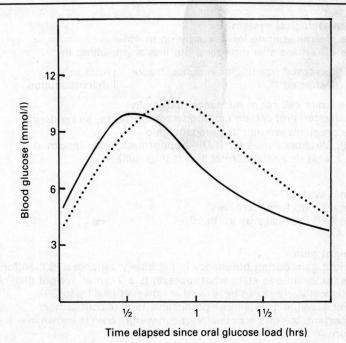

Fig. 38 Glucose tolerance curves in pregnant (dotted line) and non-pregnant women (solid line)

Adrenal function
Glucocorticoid and mineralocorticoid secretion are both increased in pregnancy.

Cardiovascular System
Cardiac output increases by approximately 30% in the first trimester, and then remains reasonably constant until term. Most of the increased output goes to the:

> uterus
> kidneys
> skin

Blood pressure changes relatively little.

Peripheral resistance drops; venous pressure increases in the lower limbs (pelvic mass effect) but not elsewhere; veins dilate.

The ECG becomes modified, mainly as a result of the heart being pushed upwards and laterally by the growing uterus, commonly resulting in:

left axis deviation
Q waves and inverted T waves in lead III
(usually reversible on deep inspiration)
ST changes in some leads

Haematological system
The plasma volume increases by up to 45%
The RBC mass also increases, but less so, resulting in:

decreased haemoglobin concentration } due to
decreased PCV   } haemodilution

The white cell count increases marginally
Fibrinogen and certain clotting factors increase, so rendering
the pregnant woman 'hypercoagulable'
N.B. Virchow's triad for DVT — abnormal blood, abnormal
     vessels and abnormal flow is thus fulfilled.

Renal system
Renal blood flow increases
The GFR increases by up to 60%

Weight gain
Weight gain during pregnancy is extremely variable and therefore
it is impossible to state what represents a 'normal' weight gain. A
statistical average can be arrived at however (see figure 39).
   Fetal weight gain is more predictable (and of course more
important, but less accessible): mean weight gain is shown in
figure 40.

DIAGNOSIS OF PREGNANCY

Relies on the same principles as any other diagnosis:

History	Delayed menstruation
	Breast fullness and tenderness
	Urinary tract symptoms, especially frequency
	Nausea
Examination:	Increased uterine size
	Cervical softening
	Increased breast activity, e.g. dilated superficial veins
Laboratory investigations:	Urine HCG assay (the 'standard' pregnancy test)
	Ultrasound scanning
	B sub-unit HCG (serum) for very early determination of pregnancy

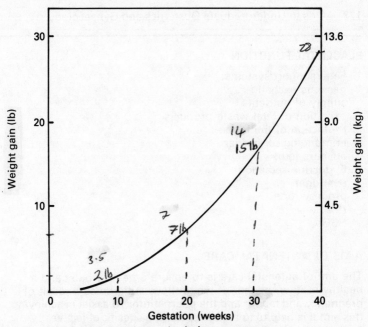

Fig. 39 Mean maternal weight gain during pregnancy

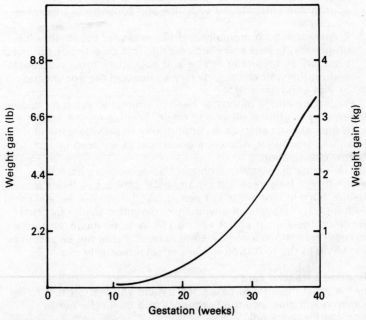

Fig. 40 Mean fetal weight gain during gestation

PLACENTAL FUNCTION

1. Fetal support systems:
   gaseous exchange
   supply of nutrients
   excretion of fetal waste products
2. Protection of the fetus:
   immunological barrier
   anchors fetus
3. Endocrine secretion:
   oestrogen
   progesterone
   HPL
   HCG

AIMS OF ANTENATAL CARE

The aim of antenatal care is to ensure a healthy baby and a
healthy mother, neither of whom have suffered as a result of
pregnancy and labour and the puerperium. To assist in achieving
this aim it is helpful to recognise certain specific objectives:
1. Prevention, detection and treatment of any disorders arising
   from or during pregnancy which threaten the wellbeing of the
   fetus and/or the mother. This objective is achieved by
   appropriate antenatal surveillance and subsequent treatment
   as indicated.
2. Preparation, both mentally and physically, of the mother for
   pregnancy, labour and child-rearing. This objective is achieved
   primarily by providing advice and education through antenatal
   and mothercraft classes, dietary advice and the administration
   of iron and folic acid.

Pregnancy brings otherwise healthy women to see their doctors
when they might not otherwise do so. For this reason antenatal
care may also be seen as an opportunity to provide general
health screening for women, e.g. cervical smear testing and
breast examination.

The perinatal mortality amongst babies who are born to
women who have received no antenatal care is five times that of
babies born to women who have received normal antenatal care.
Although this statistic is obviously confounded by the fact that
those mothers most at risk are also likely to be those least able
to 'use' antenatal services, clearly antenatal care per se accounts
for some of the reduction in the perinatal mortality rate.

Routine antenatal care

In the great majority of cases, the patient will first present to her
GP who will diagnose the pregnancy and then refer her to
hospital for 'booking'.

First hospital visit (booking clinic)
Normally done at about 10–12 weeks.

Attention is focused on	Confirming diagnosis of pregnancy
	Establishing the dating of the pregnancy
	Collecting baseline and background information
	Identification of risk factors
History:	This pregnancy
	Previous pregnancies
	Gynaecological history
	Menstrual history
	Medical history — including smoking, alcohol, drugs
	Family and social history
	Ethnic group
Examination:	Weight and height
	Blood pressure
	Urinalysis
	Cardiovascular system
	Respiratory system
	Breasts
	Abdomen
	Pelvis (including speculum)
	Teeth
	Varicose veins
Investigations:	Haemoglobin plus electrophoresis if appropriate
	ABO and Rhesus blood grouping, with antibody screen
	VDRL
	Rubella antibodies
	MSU
	HVS if appropriate
	Cervical smear
	Ultrasound scan for:
	dating the pregnancy (most accurate at 12–16 week stage)
	provision of baseline for further growth
	detection of abnormalities, e.g. multiple pregnancy

Subsequent visits
1. Frequently shared with the general practitioner.
2. Schedule of visits takes account of the fact that the frequency
   of complications increases with the duration of the pregnancy:

   monthly until 28 weeks and then ⎫ unless
   fortnightly until 36 weeks and then ⎬ otherwise
   weekly until delivery ⎭ indicated

3. Focus of attention changes as pregnancy progresses:
   (a) second trimester (usually an 'uneventful' trimester)
       (i) general assessment of fetal growth
       (ii) early detection of maternal complications including
            pre-eclampsia, anaemia, etc
   (b) third trimester
       (i) assessment of fetal maturity, growth and wellbeing
       (ii) maternal wellbeing
       (iii) mechanics of and/or possible need for intervention in
             labour
4. Clinical assessment at each visit:
   (a) weight
   (b) blood pressure
   (c) urinalysis (protein and glucose)
   (d) oedema
   (e) abdomen
       (i) uterine size
       (ii) fetal viability (fetal heart and/or movements)
       (iii) fetal lie
       (iv) fetal presentation
       (v) fetal abnormality (including amount of liquor)
       (vi) engagement of the presenting part
       (vii) abdominal examination for the position of the fetal
             back is of little value
5. Additional investigations: haemoglobin at 28 and 34 weeks
   rhesus antibodies (if appropriate) at 28 and 34 weeks
   ultrasound scans — BPD and abdominal circumference
   feto-placental function tests, e.g. serial oestriol,
   serial HPL levels
   fetal kick charts
   cardiotocographic monitoring
   The last four should be done as often as indicated.

ANTENATAL ADVICE FOR MOTHER

Consider under various headings:
1. Diet
   well-balanced
   increase protein and calcium intake
   routine iron and vitamin supplements may not be necessary

2. Habits
   stop smoking
   stop alcohol consumption
   work up until about 32 weeks if wanted
   moderate amount of exercise, plenty of rest
   sex: couples' own inclinations are the best guide unless
   medical indications override
3. Dental Care
   gingivitis very common in pregnancy — advise patient to see
   her dentist
4. General advice
   talk to the mother and answer questions
   refer to mothercraft/relaxation classes
   arrange tours of delivery suites/lectures, etc
5. Drugs
   In general, avoid prescribing in pregnancy especially in the
   first trimester (organogenesis).
   Some drugs are thought to be safe:
      antiemetics — some are safe
      antibiotics — penicillins and cephalosporins
      anticoagulants — heparin acceptable, oral anticoagulants
         less safe
      sedatives and tranquillizers — generally 'safe' (but
         thalidomide was a tranquillizer thought to be safe for use in
         pregnancy) but if used at term can cause neonatal
         respiratory depression
      antihypertensives — methyldopa, labetalol.

HIGH RISK SITUATIONS

Certain groups of pregnant women are recognised as being 'high-risk'.

Elderly primigravidae

Age greater than 35 at first pregnancy (note that it is the age
rather than the nulliparity that matters) at risk because/from:
   increased incidence of fetal abnormality the baby is likely to be
   'precious':
      previous infertility is common and available time for future
      pregnancies is limited

Special measures: amniocentesis if appropriate
                         book for hospital delivery
                         consider induction of labour at term
                         close fetal monitoring in labour

Grand multiparity

Fifth or subsequent
delivery (not
pregnancy) at risk
because/from:

increased perinatal mortality
increased maternal mortality
maternal anaemia and general ill health
unstable fetal lie, malpresentations
'precipitate' labour
late engagement of the fetal head
post-partum haemorrhage
uterine rupture

Special measures:

hospital delivery with blood available
close antenatal supervision
contraceptive advice post delivery
IV ergometrine at delivery

Obesity

at risk because/from:

increased hypertension and pre-
　　eclampsia
obstetric assessment is difficult
fat mothers produce fat (i.e. big) babies
increased operative and anaesthetic risk
increased risk of gestational DM

Special measures:

aim for no overall weight gain in
　　pregnancy
hospital delivery
glucose tolerance test
use large cuff for blood pressure
　　measurements to avoid spurious
　　overreading

Antenatal care. 2: Abnormal conditions of pregnancy

Comprehensive antenatal care has developed in order to identify those women most at risk of having an abnormal outcome to their pregnancy, i.e. those women who if left alone and unattended would suffer an increased maternal and fetal mortality and morbidity.

FETAL ABNORMALITY

Fetal abnormality may present in one or more of the following ways:

Polyhydramnios
IUGR + IUD
Breech presentation
Unstable lie
Malpresentation/abnormal lie
Disproportion
Post-maturity

Investigations

Routine:	Ultrasound
	Maternal serum alpha-fetoprotein
Special (for use when fetal abnormality is suspected):	Liquor AFP or AChE
	Chromosome analysis
	X-ray
	Fetoscopy
	Fetal blood sampling (for haemoglobinopathies)

Management

The results of all the investigations are discussed in full with the parents, who will want to be informed about many points, including the degree of handicap, the length of survival and the chance of the abnormality recurring. They are given the option of continuing with or terminating the pregnancy.

Methods of termination of pregnancy
Prostaglandin TOP using a solution or gel extra-amniotically, or a
solution + urea intra-amniotically
Hysterotomy
Some surgeons will terminate vaginally (by suction TOP) up to 18
weeks; 12 weeks is a more normal limit
  Genetic counselling should be offered to all couples who have
had an abnormal baby. They can then be advised whether the
abnormality is a 'one off' occurrence or whether there is an
increased risk of recurrence. 1 in 200 live births have
chromosomal abnormalities.
  Amniocentesis should be offered to all women over the age of
36 years, but the mother must be advised that the procedure
carries a risk of causing an abortion (variously assessed as
0.5–2.0%) and of causing fetal injury.

Down's syndrome
Incidence: 1 in 160 live births
Mothers >40 years have a 1 in 50 chance of having a Down's
  baby, rising to 1 in 20 at 45 years.
1 in 100 chance of a second Down's baby.

Spina bifida
1 in 300 risk of spina bifida, but 1 in 25 if a previous child was
  affected.
Amniocentesis gives a 90% overall pick-up for neural tube defects
  (NTD).
Ultrasound scanning is very accurate at detecting NTDs and has
  replaced serum AFP testing in some centres.

ANTEPARTUM HAEMORRHAGE

Antepartum haemorrhage is bleeding occurring from the genital
tract after 28 weeks gestation. It is serious and may lead to the
death of the mother, the baby or both. APH occurs in 5–10% of
pregnancies.

Types: 30% incidence each { Unavoidable (inevitable) (Pl. praevia)
                                 { Accidental (Abruptio placenta)
                                 { Incidental (Local)

Unavoidable
Bleeding from an abnormally situated placenta, i.e. placenta
praevia.

Features: 1 in 200 births
                       More common in multipara

Four degrees of placenta praevia used to be described depending on whether or not the placenta reached or covered the os.

From a practical viewpoint the placenta in placenta praevia is now described as:

Being in the lower segment but not covering the internal os
Partially covering the os
Completely covering the os

Accidental
Bleeding from a normally situated placenta; also called abruptio placenta. It may become apparent externally (i.e. revealed — 80%), or there may be no vaginal loss (i.e. concealed — 20%).

Incidental
Bleeding from any other genital tract lesion, e.g. polyp, erosion.

Aetiology
Unavoidable/placenta praevia
Idiopathic
LSCS scar
? poor blood supply to part of uterine body
Large placenta (twins)
Abnormal placenta (diffuse, or succenturate lobe)

Separation may be due to
Mechanical forces (labour)
Placentitis
Rupture of engorged venous lakes

Accidental
Unknown, but . . . . . .
? External version
? Fetal movements
? Increased incidence with:
   PET
   DM
   Renal disease
   Chronic hypertension

Pathophysiology
Bleeding → hypovolaemic shock
Couvelaire uterus
Disseminated intravascular coagulopathy
Acute cor pulmonale (due to amniotic cellular emboli or defibrination in the pulmonary micro-circulation)
Acute renal necrosis
Acute pituitary necrosis (Sheehan's syndrome)

Signs and symptoms

Unavoidable:
(Pl. praevia)

Spotting in 1st and 2nd trimester
PAINLESS profuse bleeding
Unengaged presenting part
10% have initial cramping
Uterus soft
Abnormal lie
Ultra-sound = placenta in lower segment

Accidental:

Uterus PAINFUL and tender
Uterus irritable
+ or — fetal distress
+ or — bleeding
Maternal shock

Management
Treatment should be commenced immediately and efficiently.

Domiciliary
Keep patient at rest, quiet and flat on left side.

Record observations
fully:

Pulse
BP
General condition
Fetal heart
Vaginal loss

Call Obstetric Flying Squad
On *NO* account do a rectal or vaginal examination.

Hospital treatment
IVI: blood (O Rh — ve if desperate) or plasma
Haemoglobin estimation
Cross-match blood
FDP estimation
Serum fibrinogen level
VERY GENTLE speculum examination to exclude lower genital
   tract bleeding (facilities for an immediate LSCS must be available)
Ultrasound scan if available on labour ward, or if the time is
   available with conservative management.
Accurate diagnosis of the cause of bleeding can be very difficult.

Further management is by clinical situation

APH of unknown cause at or near term
Perform examination under anaesthetic ('EUA') or examination
without anaesthetic ('EWA') depending on the clinical suspicion
in theatre with facilities for immediate LSCS available. If placenta
is felt (it feels 'boggy'), proceed to LSCS; if no placenta felt,
perform ARM to induce labour.

Unavoidable (placenta praevia)
Conservative

Cross-match weekly

Await the cessation of bleeding if the loss is light and there is no
  fetal distress. *Bed rest for 2-3d post bleeding*
Before 32 weeks gestation it is important to gain time for fetal
  maturity.
Low lying placentae bleed because the lower segment is 'taken
  up'. If contractions are present tocolytics may be given.
Steroids may be given if <32 weeks gestation to reduce the
  chance of the fetus developing respiratory distress syndrome
  (RDS).

Surgical
Lower segment Caesarian section (Because it may be necessary
to cut through the placenta, there is a risk of severe fetal
haemorrhage as well as the ever-present risk of major
haemorrhage to the mother.)

Accidental
Conservative
Constant maternal and fetal monitoring. Both patients are at great
risk, and the first evidence of renewed bleeding may be maternal
shock and/or loss of the fetal heart.

Surgical
Induction of labour by artificial rupture of the membranes, (ARM)
  + syntocinon
Patients with an accidental APH will often labour well.
LSCS
Caesarean section may be required in both these conditions
  even if the fetus is dead to save the mother.

RHESUS DISEASE (HAEMOLYTIC DISEASE OF THE NEWBORN)

Rhesus incompatibility may develop when a Rhesus negative
woman is impregnated by a Rhesus positive man and a Rhesus
positive fetus is conceived.

Aetiology
Rhesus +ve fetal RBCs enter the maternal circulation.
Antibody against Rhesus factor (D) is formed.
Anti-D antibodies cross the placenta.
Anti-D antibodies cause lysis of fetal RBCs.

Features
Fetal anaemia
Oedematous (hydropic) fetus
Fetal death in utero
Post-natal accumulation of fetal bilirubin
Kernicterus
First pregnancy rarely affected

Prevention

Injection of anti-D gamma-globulin within 72 hours of delivery, abortion or TOP in Rh −ve mothers.

Screening of the mother at ante-natal booking for blood group, Rhesus factor and antibodies.

Antibody titres at 28 and 34 weeks.

The development of Rhesus haemolytic disease may be detected by:

  Rising anti-D litres.

  Liquor bilirubin levels.

Treatment

Early delivery (after 32 weeks if possible)

In utero fetal transfusion to correct the anaemia

Atraumatic delivery and third stage (to reduce the feto-maternal transfusion)

After delivery (to the infant):

  Exchange transfusion

  Phototherapy

PRE-ECLAMPTIC TOXAEMIA (PET) AND ECLAMPSIA

PET is a disorder, the pathological basis of which is poorly understood, which is recognised clinically by:

  Raised blood pressure

  Oedema (or excess weight gain)

  Albuminuria

N.B. These are physical signs.

There are no symptoms of mild or moderate PET.

Of these signs, raised blood pressure is essential to the diagnosis, whilst oedema and proteinuria may or may not be present.

PET is a disease of the second half of pregnancy, and with the rare exception of molar pregnancy, should not be diagnosed before 20 weeks. It is more likely that renal disease will be responsible.

Incidence

About 5% of all pregnancies

Increased in primigravidae

May be superimposed upon hypertension

Associated with: Twins (2–3 times more common)

  Diabetes mellitus

  Hydrops fetalis

  Hydatidiform mole (This is the only situation in which PET can develop before 20 weeks).

Handwritten annotations: >110 Twice / Once

Diagnosis
Any BP >140/90 mmHg. This is an 'absolute' diagnosis.
A rise in the diastolic pressure of >20 mmHg from the pre-
pregnancy/booking levels. This is a 'relative' diagnosis.

Classification
Mild (mildly raised BP alone)
Moderate (raised BP + oedema +/or albuminuria)
Severe (eclampsia may be imminent — v.i.). At this stage the
disease becomes symptomatic.

Severe PET
Features: Headaches
                             Spots before the eyes
                             Diplopia
Examine   Dizziness
Eyes - Papilloedema   Epigastric discomfort
Reflexes - Hyperreflexia   Vomiting
                             Itchy nose

These symptoms indicate imminent eclampsia and must be
urgently treated.
    However some patients are brought in as emergencies having
had an eclamptic episode at home completely 'out of the blue'.
    Remember that most eclamptic episodes occur in the
puerperium.

Aetiology
This is unknown. It is called the disease of theories' as so many
have been advanced to explain it. Relevant factors are thought to
include:
A deficiency of prostacyclin.
Reduced refractoriness to the pressor effects of angiotensin II
Micro-emboli of trophoblast into the pulmonary circulation
Placental blood vessel changes + placental degeneration
? A failure of immune tolerance between the feto-placental unit
and the mother
Altered renal function due to a renal vascular lesion
Reduced GFR
DIC and fibrin deposition
Reduced volume in the intra-vascular compartment.

Effect on the Fetus and placenta
In utero growth retardation
In utero death
Fetal distress during labour
Fetal asphyxia

Placental changes: Infarction
                   Fibrosis replacing blood vessels
Raised perinatal mortality rate
Prematurity due to the natural onset of pre-term labour or
iatrogenic pre-term delivery

Management
Mild and moderate PET
Good antenatal care
Investigate 1st trimester hypertension
Rest
Sedation (of doubtful use)
Watch weight and salt intake
Induction of labour may be indicated in the interests of the fetus.
There is no point in allowing labour to go beyond 38–40 weeks.

Severe fulminating PET
The threat of eclampsia is prominent here, therefore:
    Heavy sedation (diazepam i.v.)
    Hydralazine or labetalol i.v.
    Induction or LSCS

Complications of severe PET/eclampsia
Accidental APH
Fetal and/or maternal death

Urinary Suppression
Patients with moderate PET have altered renal function, and in
those with severe PET oliguria may be a marked feature; tubular
or cortical necrosis may occur.

Management
Encourage diuresis post-delivery (mannitol or frusemide)
Fluid restriction
Accurate fluid balance
Continue anti-hypertensive therapy
Continue sedation.

Eclampsia
The word 'eclampsia' means to strike forth or suddenly appear,
but in fact eclampsia is the end result of a gradually progressive
disease: pre-eclamptic toxaemia. In eclampsia, the mother has
generalised convulsions, but may also be deeply comatose.
Untreated, death of the mother and fetus may result.

Incidence
Approximately 1.2–2.6/1000 deliveries
Approximately 1/200 cases of PET
Maternal mortality worldwide: 0–17%
Fetal mortality worldwide: 10–37%
   Prevention of eclampsia by adequate management of PET, including elective early delivery, is of paramount importance.
   Should eclampsia develop, it is a medical emergency which must be given the highest priority by the obstetric and midwifery team on site.

Management
The aim is to prevent maternal complications and to deliver a healthy baby:
   Establish IVI
   Give immediately diazepam 10 mg i.v.
   Repeat if necessary
   Give hydralazine i.v. by side drip to control blood pressure
   Ensure control of airway: padded spatula in mouth. Replace with
      plastic airway after convulsion
   Mother in Trendelenberg position
   Aspirate secretions/vomitus
   Estimate FBC, PCV, U+Es
   Maintain accurate fluid balance chart
   Assess the cervix: is it ripe for induction/does it suggest that the
      mother will deliver quickly?
   If cervix unfavourable, deliver fetus by LSCS
* Delivery/termination of the pregnancy is THE treatment for
PET/eclampsia.
After delivery: Continue sedation
                Practise fluid restriction
                Encourage diuresis prn with frusemide
                If coma persists, mannitol, (an osmotic diuretic)
                   may be required
                Continue accurate fluid balance
                Continue or institute anti-hypertensive treatment
                Check renal function
The authors appreciate that the management listed above may not be the same as practised at many teaching hospitals. Some prefer to use infusions of heminevrin for sedation, but caution is required here not to over-infuse the patient. At some hospitals routine checks are made to exclude the onset of a disseminated intravascular coagulopathy.
   As emphasised in the introduction, get to know the management at *your* hospital and be able to explain the discuss it.

NAUSEA AND VOMITING

This is common in pregnancy and is a sign of pregnancy. It may be due to:

HCG

Oestrogen

Oesophageal reflux (hiatus hernia)

Treatment
Promethazine (Phenergan) (Avomine 1 T̄ tds)
Antacids
Small frequent meals

HYPEREMESIS GRAVIDARUM

Intractable vomiting severe enough to cause maternal dehydration and acidosis in pregnancy.

Features
Pregnant
Vomiting
Starvation (because of nausea)
Dehydration
Keto-acidosis due to starvation
Liver damage (occasionally)
Weight loss

Management

Exclude:	Liver disease (LFTs, etc)
	Renal disease
Treatment:	i.v. fluids
	Correct electrolyte disturbance
	Parenteral vitamins
	Small bland meals
	Terminate pregnancy (very rare)

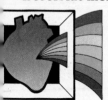

ELANTAN® 20 & 40

isosorbide mononitrate

Effective in a broad spectrum of angina patients[1,2].

Preterm Labour 28 - 37 w

25 - 34 weeks ROM / No need for Dexamet
Await Labour
Antibiotics
No need for Dexamet

34 - 37 weeks ROM / 24 hrs Postn 4
Wait for spont labour
Interswite ō no PV. for 1 week

32 - 34 ROM / To ? Det hosp. ō allow
Labour to run.
No dexameth.

(25 ROM. - Pulmonary hypoplasia
ō no liquor for 3-4 weeks

No ROM
>37 - Onwards.
34-37 - ~~Ritodrine~~ Onward.
32-34 - Cx<4cm Ritodrine. Dexamet
no harm.
28-32 - Dexameth. Rit.

No Rit for Thyrotoxicosis / ~~Heart~~ (Heart
problems.
PET / APH (by relaxing uterus)

POLYHYDRAMNIOS

In the first half of pregnancy amniotic fluid is a transudate from the maternal plasma across the membranes. In the second half of pregnancy, fetal urine is added. A volume of greater than 2000 ml equals hydramnios.

Volume
10 weeks — 30 ml
20 weeks — 350 ml
30 weeks — 1000 ml
After 38 weeks the volume declines

Composition
SG 1.008
pH 7.2
Desquamated fetal cells
Proteins (1/10 fetal serum values)
Electrolytes similar to maternal plasma

Function
Protection from injury
Maintains temperature
Allows free movement
Prevents fetal adherence to the membranes

The fetus drinks about 400–500 ml per day and excretes about the same amount.

If the drinking is interfered with (either prevented or reduced) or there is an increased urine output, hydramnios will develop.

Causes of Hydramnios
NTD
Oesophageal atresia
Duodenal atresia
Imperforate anus
Other fetal abnormality
Maternal diabetes mellitus
Multiple pregnancy

Complications (mainly due to overdistension of the uterus)
Pain
Pre-term rupture of the membranes
Pre-term labour
Abnormal lie/malpresentation

Treatment
Rest
Moral support
Analgesia
Antacids prn
Terminate pregnancy if fetal abnormality

OLIGOHYDRAMNIOS

Oligohydramnios means that there is too little liquor for the stage
of pregnancy.

Cause
Fetal urinary tract abnormality:

> Renal agenesis
> Posterior urethral valves

PRETERM RUPTURE OF THE MEMBRANES   *28 - 37 weeks*

This is spontaneous rupture of the membranes before 37 weeks
gestation.

Aetiology
- Idiopathic
- Cervical infection + infection of the adjacent membranes
  (antenatal vaginal examinations are thought to increase the risk
  of this)
- Hydramnios

Management
This <u>depends on</u> the <u>gestation</u>, the <u>fetal presentation</u> and the
presence or absence of <u>maternal pyrexia</u> (indicating amnionitis).

Ritodrine + Antibiotics (No Doxamath)

<u>After 32 weeks</u>   *To ICBU hospital*

Some would use Prostin after 24hrs but risk of LSCS.

(a) Cephalic presentation: Perform CTG: If there is fetal distress
    deliver by LSCS *or frank breech.*
    No fetal distress: await spontaneous vaginal delivery *c̄ no PV for 1 we*
    If there is a maternal pyrexia, induce contractions with *Prostin ±*
    syntocinon, or if the cervix is unfavourable, deliver by LSCS.
(b) Any other presentation:
    Deliver by LSCS (but allow frank breech to labour)

<u>Before 32 weeks</u>   *25 - 32 weeks*   *To ICBU hospital*
(a) Apyrexial:
No vaginal examination
Steroids to stimulate fetal surfactant production) *(Not Mr. Melville)*
Low vaginal swab *- Antibiotics if necessary*
Bed rest
Aim to get to 32 weeks
Tocolytics as required *i.e. Ritodrine*

<25 weeks Preserve pregnancy for as long as possible c̄
no VE, but after ~3weeks, pulmonary hypoplasia
→RDS.   Need >500g foetus for survival.

Contraindications for Ritodrine :-
PET ; Cardiac problems ; APH ; Thyrotoxicosis

(b) Pyrexial:
Cephalic: stimulate contractions if cervix ripe or LSCS if not
Breech: LSCS
Fetal distress: LSCS

PRETERM LABOUR   *28 – 37 weeks*

The onset of labour before 37 weeks gestation. Technically,
before 28 weeks, effacement and dilatation of the cervix indicate
a threatened abortion, but with modern neonatal intersive care 26
weeks is a better cut-off point.

Statistics
7% of all pregnancies
Fetus < 1500 g most at risk (up to 85% neonatal mortality)

Causes of preterm labour
Idiopathic
Urinary tract infection
Multiple pregnancy
Hydramnios
Maternal infection/pyrexia
Surgery
Injury
Iatrogenic, as in preterm delivery for:
   PET
   Renal disease
   Rhesus disease
   Placenta praevia
Cervical incompetence

Prevention
Antenatal care
Shirodkar suture (for cervical incompetence) *(Macdonald)*
Screen for urinary tract infection and treat energetically if
detected

Treatment
Tocolytic drugs
e.g. Ritodrine ⎤
   Isoxuprine ⎬ beta-sympathomimetic drugs
   Salbutamol ⎦
   Alcohol
Treat UTI if present
  If one cannot prevent preterm labour the main problem is how
to deliver the preterm fetus.

Vaginal delivery imposes considerable stress on the fragile preterm fetus. The cranial contents are especially prone to damage, and for this reason the relatively atraumatic (for the fetus) delivery by Caesarean section may be better. Cut-off points are controversial but current opinion may be summarised as follows:

Cephalic presentation; deliver by LSCS up to 1500 g/30 weeks
Breech presentation: deliver by LSCS up to 2000 g/33 weeks*

32-34   Cx <4cm   Ritodrine + Dexamethasone
28-32   "   "   "

INTRA-UTERINE GROWTH RETARDATION

This may be defined as being present when the fetal weight is less than the fifth centile for the gestational age. Although the fetus cannot be weighed in utero, the weight may be estimated from charts after measuring the bi-parietal diameter and the abdominal circumference ultrasonically. *+ Crown-rump length?*

BPD
AC

Approximately 30–40% of low birth weight babies demonstrate IUGR. If on measuring the BPD and AC both values are reduced, symmetrical IUGR, (which is early in onset) is diagnosed.

If the BPD is within the normal range for the gestational age but the AC is low, then asymmetrical IUGR is diagnosed, which is usually of late onset.

Aetiology
Maternal

Poor nutrition
Smoking
Genetic/racial features

Feto-placental

Fetal abnormality
Multiple pregnancy
Uteroplacental insufficiency due to:
PET
Placental infarcts
Placental thrombosis
Renal hypertension

Management

Hospitalisation and rest
Try to identify cause
Correct if possible
Consider preterm delivery if the cause is
  untreatable and progressive

* Based on published figures from Hammersmith Hospital, London

MULTIPLE PREGNANCY

Definition: more than one fetus is present.

Incidence

Twins 1 in 80 pregnancies
Triplets 1 in 80^2 = 1 in 6400
Quads 1 in 80^3 = 1 in 51200

Aetiology

Monozygotic pregnancies
Rate 4 per 1000
Same in all races
Not influenced by any known maternal
    factors

Dizygotic pregnancies
UK rate 12 per 1000
Probably inherited
More common in older multipara
Peak incidence 35–40 years
Increased incidence with induction of
    ovulation *(eg. Clomiphere which stimulates
    -ve feedback by gonadotrophin
    release by ting -ve feedback)*

Pathological Complications

Maternal:
Anaemia
Marked uterine distension
Increased incidence of placenta praevia

Fetal:
Twins may be small for dates
Increased incidence of congenital
    abnormality
Fetus papyraceus
Increased incidence of velamentous cord
    insertion

Multiple pregnancy is at high risk for:

Anaemia
PET/eclampsia
Haemorrhage (ante- and post-partum)
Uterine inertia
Cord prolapse
Premature separation of the placenta
Preterm labour
Twin to twin transfusion

Symptoms and signs
Exaggerated symptoms of normal pregnancy

Clinical diagnosis possible in about 75% of cases:
    palpation >3 poles
                multiple small parts
    auscultation 2 fetal hearts
    excess weight gain that is not oedema or obesity
    polyhydramnios
    palpation of 2nd fetus in uterus after delivery of the first infant

Additional investigations
Ultrasound scanning
Plain abdominal X-ray
Expect high HPL titres

Differential diagnosis
Single pregnancy, innaccurate dates
Polyhydramnios
Abdominal tumours (fibroids, ovarian cyst)

Management
Early diagnosis of multiple pregnancy
More frequent antenatal visits
More rest after 24 weeks
Hospital delivery
If possible convert second twin to cephalic presentation by
    external version after delivery of the first
Deliver the second twin as quickly as possible
May need tocolytics to delay labour (increased incidence of pre-
    term labour)
Paediatricians present at delivery
Caesarean section for obstetric reasons only
No Shirodkar suture
Frequent USS checks on both twins growth rate

BREECH   *Abnormal after 32 weeks*
A breech presentation means that the fetal buttocks ± the feet
comprise the presenting part.

Types   Incomplete or frank breech: extended
                                legs
                           Complete breech: knees flexed; feet
                                above buttocks
                           Footling breech: one or both feet below
                                buttocks
                           Knee presentation: one or both knees
                                below buttocks

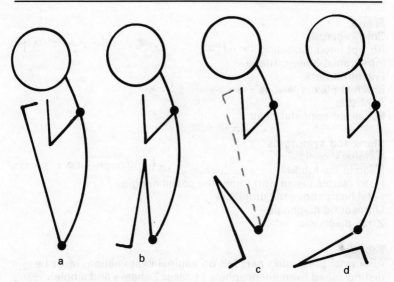

Fig. 41 The different positions of the fetus in breech presentation.
(a) Frank breech (extended breech); (b) flexed breech; (c) footling breech;
(d) knee presentation

The sacrum is used as the denominator, e.g. right sacrum
anterior, left sacro-lateral, etc.

Incidence
3% *at 36 weeks.*
Varies inversely with birth weight: higher when the birth weight
is lower

Aetiology   *Prematurity*
Maternal   Placental site — *Placenta praevia*
                       Septate/bicornuate uterus
                       Increased uterine tone
                       Oligohydramnios / *Polyhydramnios*
                       ~~Placenta praevia~~, *fibroids*

Fetal   Large head (hydrocephaly; goitre)
                       Splinting legs discourage turning, *extended at knees*
                       Twins

Pathology/dangers
Breech presentation is not especially dangerous to the mother
but is very dangerous to the fetus because of:
Failure of the presenting part to conform to the lower segment
resulting in delay in labour and uterine incoordination
Greater need for vaginal manipulation

*Head comes last and if the breech has taken a long
time to deliver, the head will take longer. It may
occlude the cord & placenta may separate → anoxia → breath → water of
blood incase*

Fetal
Cord prolapse
Abrupt head moulding *& release → cerebral haemorrhage*
Intracranial haemorrhage
Fractured neck
Brachial plexus lesions *+ sternomastoid lesions*
Asphyxia
Increased neonatal death
Hypoxia → cerebral haemorrhage

Signs and symptoms
Antenatal clinic
Head in the fundus *i.e. Palpation Retarder chin can prevent ballot*
Head causes discomfort under the costal margin
Fetal heart above the umbilicus
Ultrasound diagnosis
X-ray diagnosis

Labour
Abnormal presenting part felt on vaginal examination. Must be distinguished from anencephaly (+ face: 2 cheeks and a hole ...)
Slow labour
N.B. When palpating the breech vaginally, it is important NOT to try to insert a finger into the anus or vagina, although it is classically described that the way to distinguish the anus from the lips in a face presentation is to palpate the alveolar ridge in the latter.
    Feet are recognised by the short stubby toes, and distinguished from hands by the fact that one cannot 'shake hands' with them.

Management *Placental sep^n; Cord entanglement, ROM.*
Antenatal
External cephalic version is practised by some consultants *34/40*
Clinical X-ray pelvimetry prn *(Vaginal delivery cannot proceed without this)*
In labour
Primigravida: consider LSCS
Breech + any other abnormality (X factor) = LSCS
IVI
Cross match blood
Epidural
Monitor fetus and the labour very closely
Types of delivery *3 8/40 - smaller & head moulds easily then.*
✓ Assisted breech
High + natural Spontaneous breech
Breech extraction
Forceps to after-coming head

\Not in Hypertens due to abruptio placenta.
Multiple pregnancy
Congenital malform.
IUP
Scar

Denominator is sacrum.

Breech only 3/4 dilates cx, so mother wants to push too early for bigger head which is then held back. Epidural eliminates this (or gas for transitional stage). Do a VE to confirm dilatation before allowing the pt. to push.
§Burns Marshall manoeuvre - forceps allow slow delivery of head.
§Mauriceau - Smellie - Veit manoeuvre.

but not to mother

Breech presentation constitutes a risk to the fetus, and some obstetricians consider breech presentation to be a malpresentation and therefore feel that there is no place for a trial of breech labour or for artificial rupture of the membranes. In labour the progress must be constantly monitored, and if the cervix is not dilating at the optimal rate and the presenting part is not descending then Caesarean section should be performed without delay, even if the cervix has got to full dilatation.

UNSTABLE LIE

In this condition the fetal position keeps changing. This is normal in the first and second trimesters but puts the fetus at risk in the third trimester as there is the constant risk of cord prolapse (at the onset of labour).
    Fetal death and uterine rupture may also occur.

Causes
Idiopathic
Grand multiparity
Hydramnios
Fetal abnormality
Placenta praevia

Management
Admit to hospital at 34 weeks
If labour occurs with malpresentation: LSCS
If the lie stabilises, induce at term
If unstable at term: LSCS
(Stabilising induction in the Third World may avoid LSCS)

ABNORMAL LIE

Definition: the long axis of the fetus is not parallel to the long axis of the uterus. The lie may be:
    Transverse
    Oblique cephalic or breech

Causes
Idiopathic
Hydramnios
Fetal abnormality
Grand multiparity
Placenta praevia
Pelvic tumours
Uterine abnormality

Management
Antenatal: observe. Admit at 34 weeks gestation
In labour or at term: deliver by Caesarean section

DISPROPORTION

Cephalopelvic disproportion exists when the diameters of the pelvis are smaller than the presenting diameters of the fetal head. The matter is not as clear cut as it sounds because of moulding of the fetal head in labour, and 'relaxation' of the maternal joints at delivery.

Aetiology
Maternal
Small woman with small pelvis
Pelvic tumours reducing the pelvic diameters
Contracted pelvis: Congenital
                    Rickets
                    Fracture/injury

Fetal
Occipito-posterior positions
Large baby (DM; hydrops fetalis)
Abnormal presentations (brow or face)
Hydrocephaly

Management
Suspect antenatally (high head)
Trial of labour (cross-match blood ready for LSCS if required)
Head descends (anticipate vaginal delivery)
No cervical dilatation or descent of the head in the presence of good contractions = Caesarean section

Post-Caesarean section
X-ray pelvimetry

FETAL ALCOHOL SYNDROME

Alcohol is a drug which passes easily across the placenta. In the past it has been thought that a moderate intake of alcohol in pregnancy had no adverse effects on the fetus or uterus.
   Infants born to chronic alcoholics show:
   Alcohol withdrawal at birth
   Low birth weight/growth retardation
   Microcephaly
   Anomolies of the: face
                     eyes
                     heart
                     joints
                     external genitalia

The fetal alcohol syndrome in which the affected fetus shows some of the major features listed above, has been described in 26% of fetuses born to women who were considered alcoholics.

Expert opinion is divided as to the effect that lighter alcohol intakes have on the fetus. In one British investigation an intake of 10 single drinks per week was associated with an increased risk of delivering a low birth weight baby. Smaller amounts of alcohol have not been established to be safe.

N.B. Alcohol has a tocolytic action if the membranes are intact.

IUD   Vaginal delivery

Safe to leave 4-5 weeks, then DIC because thromboplastins enter maternal circulation leading to fibrin deposition.

Use every available induction method:

Prostin pessary
Extra amniotic prostaglandins
Syntocinon
Foley catheter via cx c̄ balloon inflated

NB. Not intra amniotic prostin due to spasticity of liquor.

Antenatal care. 3. Medical conditions affecting pregnancy

NON PRE-ECLAMPTIC HYPERTENSION IN PREGNANCY

Incidence: 1% of all pregnancies

Definition: Blood pressure which is consistently above 140/90 mmHg which either antedates the pregnancy, or is demonstrated prior to 20 weeks gestation. The point is to exclude pregnancy induced hypertension (ie pre-eclampsia) which can be difficult as pre-eclampsia may be superimposed on chronic maternal hypertension which has not been previously diagnosed.

Causes
1. Essential (idiopathic) hypertension is most common but any of the recognised causes of hypertension may be present.
2. Examination: look especially for:
   (a) cardiac abnormality (either causing or resulting from the hypertension)
   (b) coarctation of the aorta
   (c) renal artery stenosis
   (d) retinopathy (suggestive of chronic disease)
3. Investigations:
   (a) renal function tests (don't forget urinalysis!)
   (b) urinary VMA
   (c) repeated MSUs
In general these patients will be admitted for observation and investigation, although some authorities suggest only the urinary VMA (to exclude phaeochromocytoma) need be performed, all other investigations being deferred until after the pregnancy.

Complications and consequences:
1. Effects of the disease on pregnancy and the fetus:

  (a) increased perinatal mortality (×.2 if diastolic greater than 100 mmHg)
  (b) decreased uterine blood flow
  (c) intra-uterine growth retardation
  (d) placental abruption
2. Effects of pregnancy on the disease:
  (a) super-added pre-eclampsia
  (b) medical consequences of hypertension, e.g. CVA; renal sequelae

Management
1. Jointly with physician if necessary
2. Rest — either at home or in hospital
3. Antihypertensives — usually methyldopa, labetalol, hydralazine
4. Close monitoring of placental function and fetal growth
5. Induce delivery at 38 weeks
6. Avoid ergometrine (hypertensive effect)

PHAEOCHROMOCYTOMA

Rare but extremely serious: mortality 50–100%
  Suggested clinically by severe intermittent hypertension but is easily missed and urinary VMA estimation is essential in all pregnant patients in whom hypertension is diagnosed, and postnatally

Complications and consequences
1. Effects of disease on pregnancy and fetus:
  (a) increased placental abruption
  (b) maternal and fetal death
2. Effects of pregnancy on disease:
  (a) frequency and severity of hypertensive episodes are increased
  (b) greatly increased maternal mortality

Treatment
Tumour removal is the only acceptable treatment, no matter what stage pregnancy is at.

DIABETES

Incidence: the incidence of pregnant diabetics is increasing as improved general diabetic control improves fertility

Detection and diagnosis

1. If routine urinalysis reveals (a) heavy glycosuria (2%) on one occasion or (b) any glycosuria on two occasions an oral GTT should be performed. The other causes of glycosuria should not be forgotten:
   - (a) renal glycosuria (low renal threshold)
   - (b) alimentary glycosuria (rapid gut absorption causes high blood levels which exceed normal renal threshold)
2. A GTT should also be performed on any woman with a history suggestive of diabetes:
   - (a) previous large babies (greater than 9 lb)
   - (b) previous unexplained stillbirth/neonatal death
   - (c) family history of diabetes
   - (d) marked obesity during or following a previous pregnancy
   - (e) congenital abnormality
3. However, up to 30% of gestational diabetics do not have any features suggestive of diabetes and it has been suggested that all pregnant women should have a modified/short GTT.

Complications and consequences

1. Effects of diabetes on pregnancy and fetus:
   - (a) rapid fetal growth causes large baby with attendant problems
   - (b) increased intra-uterine death (particularly late on), fetal abnormality and premature labour
   - (c) increased polyhydramnios
   - (d) increased neonatal RDS ($\times$ 5) and hypoglycaemia
   - (e) increased pre-eclampsia
   - (f) increased maternal infections including pyelonephritis, vulvo-vaginal candidiasis.
2. Effects of pregnancy on disease:
   - (a) pregnancy may be considered diabetogenic (for a number of reasons) particularly as it may precipitate exposure of a latent diabetic. The figure illustrates the different types of diabetics encountered in obstetrics.

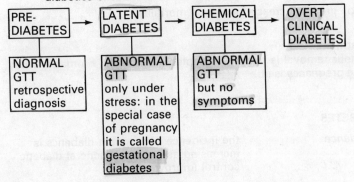

   (b) insulin requirements increase; diabetic control becomes more difficult

   (c) renal threshold for glucose drops from about 4 months meaning urine testing cannot be reliably used to monitor diabetic control

Management

1. Good management reduces maternal and fetal risks to near normal and ideally starts in a pre-conception clinic.
2. Should be undertaken in specialist units.
3. Insulin should be increased as requirements increase.
4. Monitor by blood sugar (not urine — see above).
5. Maternal glycosylated haemoglobin levels useful for assessing quality of control.
6. Treat any intercurrent illness, especially infection, early and vigorously.
7. Frequent monitoring of feto-placental unit.
8. Induce labour, either at 38 weeks, or, if control good and no obstetric contraindication to waiting, at term.
9. Early recourse to Caesarean section if required.
10. Neonatal paediatrician should be in attendance at delivery.
11. Following delivery, the mother normally returns to her pre-pregnancy diabetic status.

HEART DISEASE

Incidence: less than 1% of all pregnancies. The figure is becoming even less due to the reduction in rheumatic heart disease. Majority of patients now have congenital (rather than rheumatic) heart disease.

Diagnosis

1. Best done by a physician/cardiologist.
2. Achieved through normal means: history, examination, CXR and ECG and echocardiography.
3. Allowances should be made for the hyperdynamic circulatory state present in pregnancy (increased incidence of innocent murmurs).
4. If in doubt, the patient should be managed as if she had heart disease, and re-examined 6 weeks post-natally, a definite diagnosis reached and the patient informed.

Complications and consequences

1. Effect of pregnancy on heart disease:
   (a) risk of right and/or left sided heart failure
   (b) particular risk of acute left ventricular failure in labour and immediately after due to 'autotransfusion' from the contracting uterus

   (c) risk of bacterial endocarditis
   (d) deterioration in the maternal cardiac functional disability
2. Effect of heart disease on pregnancy and fetus:
   (a) cyanotic congenital heart disease results in increased perinatal mortality
   (b) in general acyanotic and other heart disease does not adversely effect the pregnancy or fetus
   (c) fetus may inherit maternal defect if she has congenital heart disease

Management

1. Jointly with a cardiologist.
2. If cardiac failure develops admit and treat vigorously.
3. Treat concurrent disease (especially anaemia) vigorously.
4. Beware preeclampsia (imposes even greater strain on heart).
5. Allow spontaneous labour if possible and then expedite delivery, possibly with use of elective forceps.
6. Prophylactic antibiotics (controversial).
7. Avoid ergometrine and oxytocics.
8. If cardiac failure does develop, treat with:
   (a) position — sit patient up if possible
   (b) frusemide
   (c) oxygen
   (d) venesection (actual or tourniquets)
9. Consider possibility of elective mitral valvotomy during the pregnancy.

ANAEMIA

Incidence: commonest medical disorder affecting pregnancy. Incidence figures vary with definition and where study is done.

Definition

1. Pregnancy produces a state of haemodilution which may result in apparent but not true anaemia.
2. Iron (and other haematological) requirements are greatly increased in pregnancy and therefore reduced maternal stores occur commonly but without progressing to frank anaemia.
3. It is therefore difficult to say whether a low measured haemoglobin in pregnancy reflects haemodilution, true anaemia or both.
4. It is correspondingly difficult to set a lower limit of normal for the haemoglobin in pregnancy. In practice the following figures are used:
   (a) haemoglobin less than 10–11 g/dl represents anaemia
   (b) haemoglobin between 11–13 g/dl: possible anaemia, possibly haemodilution, possibly both; requires investigation and follow-up.

Causes and diagnosis

1. The causes of anaemia in pregnancy are the same as those in non-pregnant women: in this country nutritional iron deficiency anaemia is the commonest cause of anaemia in pregnancy.
2. Diagnosis is usually by routine haemoglobin estimation, but patient may also present with the classical clinical features of anaemia (especially murmurs).
3. Investigation
   (a) usually the blood film and/or indices will suggest iron deficiency which can be accepted as the diagnosis.
   (b) further investigation if required includes:
     (i) serum iron
     (ii) TIBC
     (iii) serum folate/B12
     (iv) stool for ova, cysts and parasites and occult blood
     (v) remember sickle testing in African and Asian patients
     (vi) Hb electrophoresis for haemoglobinopathies

Complications and consequences

1. Effect of disease on pregnancy and fetus:
   (a) increased perinatal mortality if Hb less than 9 g/dl
   (b) intra-uterine growth retardation
   (c) increased incidence of pre-eclampsia
   (d) less reserve for haemorrhage in or after labour
2. Effect of pregnancy on anaemia
   (a) aggravation of anaemia (haemodilution and haemorrhage)
   (b) further depletion of iron stores

Management

1. Prophylactic iron (and folic acid) from 12 weeks (if started before may increase fetal abnormality rate) but routine administration is controversial.
2. Treatment of cause if identified.
3. Parental iron is rarely needed and infusion should be avoided if possible because of the risk of precipitating cardiac failure, allergic reaction, etc.

URINARY TRACT DISEASE

Urinary tract infections

1. Pregnancy predisposes to urinary tract infection by causing atonic distended ureters which occur because of
   (a) partial ureteric obstruction by the gravid uterus
   (b) the hormones present during pregnancy (especially progesterone) cause smooth muscle relaxation
2. 6% of pregnant women have asymptomatic bacteriuria on routine investigation. Initial treatment should be with amoxycillin or equivalent.

3. Failure to treat bacteriuria or recurrence may result in acute pyelonephritis and preterm labour
   (a) varies clinically from a mild malaise to a severe infection with high pyrexia and rigors which may result in premature labour, intra-uterine death or permanent maternal renal damage
   (b) treatment:
      (i) antibiotics
      (ii) lower temperature — paracetamol, tepid sponging

Other renal disease
1. Relevance to pregnancy depends on presence or absence of associated hypertension:
   (a) hypertension present: mother and fetus subject to all the complications of hypertension in pregnancy (q.v.)
   (b) hypertension not present: little effect either on mother and fetus or on the renal disease itself
2. Investigation, diagnosis and management are the same as for non-pregnant patients.

LIVER DISEASE

Vascular spiders and palmar erythema occur in pregnancy and do not suggest liver disease, but rather reflect the high levels of circulating oestrogens.

Pathology of the liver in pregnancy is rare (and 50% of that which does occur is viral hepatitis): classification is as follows:
1. Liver disease related to pregnancy
   (a) acute fatty liver of pregnancy (very rare but usually fatal)
   (b) recurrent intrahepatic cholestasis of pregnancy (rare but usually mild disorder)
   (c) liver disease associated with hyperemesis
   (d) liver disease associated with eclampsia
2. Liver disease not related to the pregnancy (i.e. coincidental)
   (a) includes all the usual liver diseases
   (b) viral hepatitis and gall stones commonest
   (c) treatment is essentially unaltered by the pregnancy

THYROID DISEASE

Note: Apart from the FTI and free serum thyroxine, standard thyroid investigations are of little use in pregnancy because of the 'pseudohyperthyroid' state induced by the pregnancy

Simple goitre
Increased iodine requirements in pregnancy may produce a goitre or cause a pre-existent goitre to enlarge

Hyperthyroidism
1. Severe hyperthyroidism impairs fertility and is therefore rarely seen in pregnancy; if pregnancy does occur, there is an increased incidence of abortion, perinatal mortality and pre-eclampsia.
2. Grave's disease may stimulate fetal hyperthyroidism, possibly due to LATS crossing the placenta.
3. Milder degrees of hyperthyroidism properly treated result in minimal risk to mother or fetus
4. Main risk is from over-enthusiastic treatment with anti-thyroid drugs so rendering the mother hypothyroid (q.v.) and/or the fetus hypothyroid resulting in cretinism. Other treatment modalities are seldom if ever used in pregnancy.
N.B. Large fetal goitres can produce deflexion of the head leading to disproportion in labour.

Hypothyroidism
1. Impairs fertility and therefore rarely seen in pregnancy.
2. If present may cause abortion and premature labour.
3. Well-controlled patients on thyroxine will need increased thyroxine during the pregnancy.

PELVIC MASSES

Fibroids
1. Usually diagnosed in early pregnancy (if not before).
2. Complications:
   (a) pre-pregnancy — infertility
   (b) increased abortion rate
   (c) red degeneration of pregnancy: caused by obstruction to venous outflow: treatment is conservative
   (d) obstruction of labour: rare as fibroids are normally carried upwards as lower segment forms: cervical fibroids may require caesarean section (avoid myomectomy)
   (e) increased post-partum haemorrhage

Ovarian masses
1. Majority are benign
2. Complications:
   (a) may be subject to the normal complications of ovarian masses:
       (i) rupture
       (ii) torsion
       (iii) bleeding
   (b) may cause obstruction of labour
3. Management: large tumours (greater than 6–10 cm) should be removed, ideally at 16 weeks gestation.

Intrapartum care. 1: Normal delivery

Labour is the process whereby the fetus, placenta and membranes are expelled from the mother. It represents the period of greatest risk to both mother and fetus, and medical management reflects this. It is also the emotional climax of pregnancy. Modern trends to humanise labour wards reflect a new awareness of this fact.

Modern obsterics is capable of providing both safe and satisfying care for the great majority of pregnant women.

PHYSIOLOGY OF NORMAL LABOUR

Initiation
1. Not fully understood. Overcomes progesterone effect.
2. Main trigger fetal rather than maternal.
3. May involve fetal cortisol.
4. Once initiated, labour appears to be self-perpetuating.
5. Prostaglandins now thought to be involved.

Mechanism of Labour
This is the technical name for the mechanics of the process and can be divided into various parts:
1. *Descent and engagement*:
   The fetal head descends and engages the maternal pelvis, usually in the transverse diameter (i.e. in the occipitolateral position).
2. *Flexion and internal rotation*:
   Further contractions increase the flexion of the fetal head and cause further descent: as the fetal head descends, the muscles of the pelvic floor provide a 'channel' which causes the head to rotate through 90°, to bring the occiput anteriorly, so that it lies under the maternal symphysis pubis (internal rotation).
3. *Extension and delivery of the head*:
   Extension of the flexed fetal head which is by now in the lowest part of the birth canal results in its delivery.

4. *External rotation of the head and delivery of the body*:
The shoulders (which also enter the pelvis in the transverse
diameter) descend and rotate through 90° to allow their
delivery in the AP diameter. As they rotate they cause the
already delivered head to rotate through a further 90° (external
rotation/restitution.) The anterior shoulder then slides out from
under the pubis and the body is born by lateral flexion.

DIAGNOSIS STAGES AND MANAGEMENT OF LABOUR

The onset of labour is defined as the beginning of regular (i.e. at
least one every 10 minutes) painful contractions. Other associated
events may assist in the diagnosis, but are not on their own
diagnostic:
1. show — passage of blood stained mucus
2. rupture of the membranes ('waters breaking')
3. cervical dilation of greater than 2 cm
4. Cervical effacement in primigravidae

Stages of Labour
1. First stage: onset of labour to full cervical dilation
(average duration: primigravida 8–10 hr;
multigravida 6–8 hr); may be divided
into latent and active phases

2. Second stage: full cervical dilation to delivery of the
fetus: time limits may be set, often
that second stage should not last more
than 1 hour, but 80 minutes is more
realistic

3. Third stage: delivery of the fetus to delivery of the
placenta and membranes: routinely
actively managed and typically lasts
5–10 minutes

Management of Labour
The majority of patients are delivered in hospital and therefore
require:
1. Admission
2. Brief history and examination (assuming adequate ante-natal
care
3. Routine shaving and enemas are not required but a bath is
recommended

Monitoring of maternal and fetal wellbeing:
1. Maternal wellbeing:
   (a) mental state

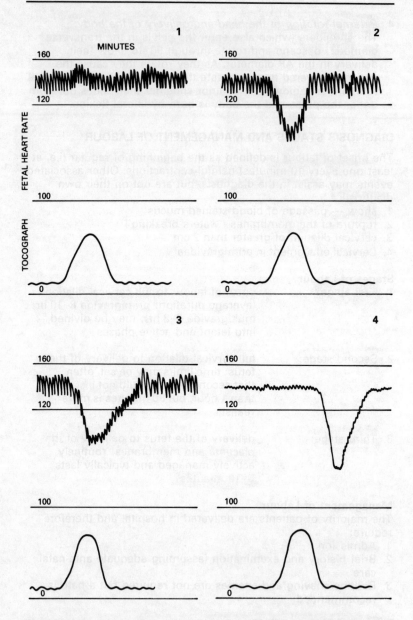

Fig. 42 (1) Normal response to a contraction; (2) early deceleration; (3) variable deceleration; (4) late deceleration and reduced beat-to-beat variability

(b) Physical state
    (i) pulse, BP and temperature
    (ii) fluid balance
    (iii) urinanalysis
(c) Progress of the labour
    (i) cervical dilation (should be approx 1 cm/hr or better)
    (ii) descent of the fetal head (assessed abdominally and vaginally
    (iii) uterine activity: frequency and duration of contractions.
2. Fetal wellbeing
  (a) fetal heart rate (monitor continuously if 'at risk' fetus for signs of distress).

      Normal cardiotocograph trace:
                    Rate 120–160/min
                    Beat-to-beat variation
                    >5/min
                    No decelerations
                    Accelerations present.
      Fetal distress indicated by:
              1. Tachycardia >160/min especially with decelerations
              2. Bradycardia <120/min and especially with decelerations
              3. Marked early decelerations
              4. Late decelerations.

  but: note that less than 50% of fetuses with a heart rate change suggestive of distress will actually have distress as assessed by Apgar score/blood pH at delivery.
  (b) meconium staining of the liquor: may be unreliable
  (c) fetal blood pH (undertaken where facilities exist if CTG abnormal)
    (i) most invasive, but also most reliable index
    (ii) fetal blood pH of less than 7.2 suggests severe

Conduct of Labour

First Stage
1. Advantages of maternal mobility and freedom from unnecessary medical monitoring are being increasingly recognised.
2. Allow bland oral fluids, but no food.
3. Oral liquid antacids every 2 hours.
4. Encourage frequent micturition.
5. Dehydration *may* require parental fluids; keto-acidosis does require parenteral fluids.
6. Allow mother to adopt her own posture.
7. Provide analgesia as required (q.v.).

Second stage
1. Allow mother to push when she wants (traditionally was only encouraged to push with contractions).
2. Monitor fetal heart rate after each contraction (if continuous trace not available).
3. Provide analgesia as required (q.v.).
4. Delivery procedure:
    (a) strict asepsis
    (b) empty bladder
    (c) usually occurs with mother semi-prone, but actual position does not matter provided the attendant:
        (i) can control the fetal head
        (ii) has access to the fetal mouth and nose (to aspirate)
        (iii) can 'protect' the maternal perineum
5. Episiotomy should be performed if indicated (q.v.).
6. Once delivered, the baby must be kept warm.
7. The cord should be cut between clamps once the pulsations have ceased.

Third Stage
1. Now virtually always actively managed.
2. Syntometrine (0.5 mg ergometrine and 5 units syntocinon) given i.m. with the anterior shoulder (N.B. Ergometrine contraindicated in hypertensive patients and some cardiac cases).
3. Await placental separation (and descent into vagina) as indicated by:
    (a) uterus becoming hard and globular
    (b) Uterus appearing to rise in abdomen
    (c) further descent of the cord (clamp placed on cord at introitus can be used as marker)
4. Deliver placenta and membranes by controlled cord traction.
5. Weigh placenta and membranes and check they are intact.
6. Estimate maternal blood loss.
7. Assess maternal condition: pulse, blood pressure, uterine size.
8. If required, carry out perineal repair as soon as possible.

EPISIOTOMY

Perineal incision under local (or general) anaesthesia to facilitate delivery. It has become a controversial procedure in normal deliveries, but there are some established indications for its use.

Indications (see note above):
1. Incipient tearing of the perineum (on the premise that a cut is easier to repair than a tear; and to avoid 3rd degree tears. Tears reported as less painful.
2. 'Rigid' perineum causing second stage delay.

3. Fetal prematurity (fetal head is especially vunerable).
4. In preparation for vaginal procedures, e.g. forceps delivery.
5. Occipito-posterior position delivery.
6. Breech delivery (especially in primigravida).
7. Previous vaginal surgery.
8. Fetal distress in 2nd stage.

Complications
1. Extension, often towards the anal margin, potentially resulting third degree tearing (avoid with 'J' shaped incision).
2. Intravaginal extension.
3. Subsequent dyspareunia.
4. Complications of any surgical procedure, in particular:
     (a) profuse haemorrhage
     (b) infection

ANALGESIA (FOR NORMAL DELIVERY)
1. Marked reductions in the need for analgesia can be achieved by natural childbirth techniques including maternal relaxation and understanding of the process of labour.
2. Drugs:
     (a) inhalational:
          (i) entonox (safe and generally available) 50% O_2/50% N_2O
          (ii) trilene
     (b) parenteral:
          (i) pethidine: widely used, especially in the first stage, but has problem that if used within 4 hours of delivery can cause neonatal respiratory depression requiring Narcan (naloxone) for reversal.
     (c) oral analgesics are generally not strong enough to merit their use
3. Anaesthesia:
     (a) general: not appropiate to normal delivery
     (b) regional: epidural anaesthesia may lead to increased forceps deliveries; pudendal block
     (c) local (field) anaesthesia: perineal infiltration with lignocaine, e.g. in preparation for episiotomy
4. 'Non-medical' analgesia:
     (a) psychoprophylaxis-very important, combined with education of the mother at antenatal classes
     (b) hypnosis

Intrapartum care. 2. Abnormal delivery

INDUCTION OF LABOUR

Induction of labour is the artificial initiation of uterine contractions by medical and/or surgical means.

Medical:
Prostaglandin E_2: (a) oral
                 (b) vaginal
Syntocinon by intra-venous infusion

Surgical:
Amniotomy (ARM: artificial rupture of the membranes) either forewaters or hindwaters
Sweeping the membranes — digital stimulation of the lower segment/cervix

Indications for induction

Although the indications for induction may be maternal or fetal, often they overlap, and here they are listed together:

Pre-eclampsia *Protein ++ & Diast >100 for >3/52 Deliver at 32 weeks*
oedema
Eclampsia
* Post-maturity
Abruptio placenta
Placental insufficiency/IUGR   *Twins:- ↑ risk placental failure of one post 38w.*
Rhesus disease
Intra-uterine death
Hydramnios
Amnionitis
Non pre-eclamptic hypertensive disorders
Diabetes mellitus
Elderly primigravidae at term
foetal distress   *Prostin + CTG & watch like hawk. Prepare for LSCS*

Contraindications

Absolute:
Placenta praevia
Abnormal lie
Known contracted pelvis

* *Post maturity 740/40   Larger baby c̄ more skull ossification*
No serious placental failure until 44 weeks
then survival = that at 36 weeks, so good.

If cx is ripe, INDUCE (<1cm long, mid posn, admits a finger, presenting part eng)
If not, CTG (foetal distress?) ✓ } leave to 43 or 44 weeks.
*   US (adequate liquor?) ✓*

Relative:	High presenting part
	Previous LSCS
	Breech presentation

Induction is likely to fail in the presence of an unripe cervix.

Bishop's score is occasionally used literally to score the ripeness of the cervix.

Ripe = cervix soft

cervical os anterior

cervix fully effaced   *or < 1 cm long*

cervical os 2 cm dilated

presenting part 1 or 2 cm below the ischial spines

Unripe (unfavourable for induction) =

cervix firm

cervical os posterior

cervix 40–50% effaced (about 2–3 cm long)

cervix closed

presenting part 1 or 2 cm above the ischial spines

It is possible to ripen the cervix (i.e. make it more favourable for induction) by giving prostaglandin E_2 tablets, pessaries or gel vaginally, or the tablets orally.

Complications	Failed induction → Caesarean section
	Fetal distress (caution when inducing for IUGR; LSCS may be better)
	Rupture of scarred uterus
	Rupture of multigravid uterus (rupture of the primigravid uterus is very rare)
	Placental detachment
	Rupture of vasa praevia
	Cord prolapse
	Amniotic fluid embolus (rare; associated with oxytocics immediately after ARM)
	Amnionitis

ABNORMAL LABOUR

Abnormal labour occurs when the process of labour is not proceeding in the normal way, i.e. the cervix is not dilating at 1 cm per hour at least, and the presenting part is not descending. Although there are many cases, this may be regarded as the 'final common pathway' which is common to all abnormal labours.

Causes (traditionally defined as a fault of one or more of the following):	The passenger
	The passages
	The powers (forces)

The passenger:	Malpresentation
	Malposition
	Hydrocephaly
	Fetal tumour
	Macrosomia (diabetic pregnancies)
	Hydrops fetalis
	Locked twins
	Siamese twins/monsters

The passages:	Pelvic tumour
	Pelvic contracture: inlet
	mid-cavity
	outlet
	Low placenta
	Cervical fibrosis/stenosis
	Vaginal septum
	Rigid perineum

| *The powers* (*force*) — inadequate: | Incoordinate uterine activity (primigravidae) |
| | Maternal exhaustion — dehydration + ketoacidosis |

TRIAL OF LABOUR

A trial of labour may be indicated where cephalo-pelvic disproportion is suspected. The obstetrician is testing the ability of the fetus to pass through the pelvis. In the past, the term trial of labour was further subdivided to be more specific about which feature was actually being tested. Thus the terms 'trial of inlet', 'trial of scar', 'trial of breech' were recorded.

Nowadays, the term trial of labour implies that the progress of labour is going to be closely assessed using the parameters of cervical dilatation and descent of the presenting part in the presence of good uterine contractions. The term implies that should labour not progress normally, the fetus will be delivered by Caesarean section.

Cephalo-pelvic disproportion
See p. 146.

Malposition
Malposition refers to abnormal positions of the occiput *in a vertex presentation*:
Occipito-posterior positions
Occipito-lateral positions (deep transverse arrest)
Occipito-posterior (*OP*)
The occiput is posterior to the pelvic transverse diameter.

Although it may be suspected before the onset of labour (non-engaged head at term), or in early labour (slow progress), many OP positions are not recognised until well into the labour.

Aetiology	
Fetal:	Extended head — goitre
	increased tone causing neck extension
Maternal:	Anthropoid pelvis
	Grande multipara — lax muscles
Pathophysiology	Poor stimulation of lower segment
	Non-engagement of head
	Delay 1st stage
	Uterine inertia
	Maternal distress
	Fetal distress
	Deep transverse arrest
	Delay 2nd stage
Signs and symptoms	
Antenatal:	Flattened abdomen/uterus
	Fetal limbs easily palpable
	Non-engaged head (especially primigravidae)
	Fetal heart loudest in flanks
In labour:	Posterior fontanelle (identified by 3 sutures) in posterior pelvis
	Severe backache
	Delay 1st stage
	Retention of urine
Management	
Antenatal:	There is nothing active that one can do except hope for normal labour with rotation to an occipito-anterior position.
In labour:	Ensure good contractions (syntocinon prn)
	Epidural analgesia
	Close fetal monitoring
	No progress 1st stage — LSCS
	No progress in 2nd stage — wide episiotomy forceps, either deliver OP or rotate with Kiellands to OA and deliver LSCS

Complications
Maternal:

Distress — emotional and metabolic
Anaesthetic hazards
Infection
Haemorrhage (vaginal vault laceration)
Thrombo-embolism
Complications of LSCS:
    wound haematoma
    UTI
    wound abscess
    ureter damage

Fetal:

Distress
Cord prolapse
Intrapartum death
Neurological damage

DEEP TRANSVERSE ARREST

The fetal head is stuck in an occipito-lateral position, in the
   transverse diameter of the outlet, between the ischial spine.
Transverse arrest may occur higher, in the mid-cavity of the pelvis.

Aetiology
Deflexion of the fetal head
Poor uterine contractions
Inadequate channelling of the fetal head by the pelvic floor (as
   happens with a relaxed pelvic floor under epidural)

Pathophysiology
As for OP positions (vs)

Management
1st Stage:

Ensure good contractions with oxytocics
If labour becomes arrested, i.e. there is
no further cervical dilatation, proceed to
Caesarian section

2nd Stage:

Kielland's rotational forceps
Ventouse (vacuum) extraction
Caesarean section

MALPRESENTATIONS

A malpresentation is any presentation other than by the vertex.
This includes:

> Breech presentation
> Brow presentation
> Face presentation
> Shoulder presentation

Brow
Incidence:
1:2000 deliveries

Diagnosis
High head
Large presenting diameter
Orbital ridges palpable
(X-ray can confirm)

Management
Vaginal examination to exclude cord prolapse
Caesarean section

A brow presentation is unstable and may spontaneously flex in labour, or may further extend to become a face presentation, which if it is mento-anterior (see below) can be delivered vaginally.

Outcome
Safest by Caesarean section, but can occasionally deliver vaginally

Face
Incidence:
1:500 deliveries

Diagnosis
High head
Orbital ridges, mouth and gums palpable + chin

Management
Determine the position of the chin, the denominator in this
   presentation
Mento-posterior and mento-lateral: Caesarean section
Mento-anterior: as for normal labour but anticipate delay and
   beware of cord prolapse. Perform a wide episiotomy and
   forceps delivery if required.
Kielland's forceps for rotation may occasionally be required.

Fetal outcome
Oedematous face
Bruised face
Sucking initially difficult

Shoulder
Incidence:
Not known

Diagnosis
Arm in the vagina on examination
Anicipate when: Transverse lie
                           Lax uterus
                           Placenta praevia (partial)
                           Multiple pregnancy
                           Hydramnios

Management
Deliver by Caesarean section

PRESENTATION AND PROLAPSE OF THE CORD

Presentation: A loop of cord lies below the presenting
                         part; the membranes are intact.

Prolapse: The cord is below the presenting part
                         and the membranes have ruptured. It
                         occurs in about 1:400 deliveries.

Aetiology
Long cord
Poorly fitting presenting part (e.g. in malpresentations)
Malposition
Hydramnios
Twins (especially the 2nd cord)

Diagnosis
The cord may be visible at the introitus
Vaginal examination

Complications
Fetal death

Management
Dead fetus: continue vaginal delivery unless
                         shoulder presentation which requires
                         either a destructive operation on the
                         fetus or a Caesarean section

Palpate cord for pulsation

Live fetus: Keep hand in the vagina
Monitor fetal heart
Keep presenting part off the cord *(buttocks on pillow)*
Raise end of the bed
Lay mother on her side
Caesarean section

If cord prolapse occurs in the second stage, a rapid forceps delivery is performed.

MULTIPLE PREGNANCY

See pp 141–142.

TECHNIQUES OF ABNORMAL DELIVERY

Forceps
Forceps deliveries either involve rotating the fetal head or they do not. The former are called rotational forceps and the latter straight forceps deliveries.

Types of forceps
Kielland's (rotational forceps)
Wrigley's (outlet/low cavity forceps)
Neville Barnes
Haigh Ferguson's
Simpson's

Indications
Delay in the 2nd stage (ensure good contractions first)
OP positions
Deep transverse arrest
Fetal distress
Maternal distress
Maternal hypertensive disorders
Maternal cardiac disorders
Maternal pulmonary disorders
After-coming head in breech

Prerequisites
Cervix fully dilated
Bladder empty
Membranes ruptured
Head must be engaged with none palpable per abdomen
Denominator must be identified
Uterine contractions must be effective
Adequate anaesthesia
Episiotomy

Anaesthesia
Perineal infiltration
Pudendal block
Caudal block
Epidural
General

Complications

Maternal:	Lacerations of genital tract (cervical tear, 3rd degree tear, etc)
	Haemorrhage
	Shock
	Retention of urine
	Failed forceps (proceeding to Caesarean section)

Fetal:	Cephalhaematoma
	Facial palsy
	Intra-cranial haemorrhage
	Bruising

Forceps delivery is attended by increased maternal and fetal mortality and morbidity. No longer are 'high' (i.e. the fetal head is high in the pelvic cavity above the ischial spines) forceps deliveries acceptable in modern British obstetric practice. Caesarean section is safer and therefore preferred.

Ventouse extraction

| Indications | As for forceps delivery |
| Prerequisites | |

Complications
Maternal
As for forceps delivery

Fetal
Cephalhaematoma (which resolves spontaneously)
Ulceration of the scalp
Tentorial tears/intracranial haemorrhage
　　Failed Ventouse extraction is an indication for Caesarean section, *not* a trial of forceps.
　　It is very important that the cup of the Ventouse is placed as close as possible to the occiput so as to assist flexion of the head.

Caesarean section
Caesarean section is the delivery of the fetus through the abdominal wall. It may be an elective or an emergency procedure.

Indications
Disproportion
Placenta praevia
Prolonged labour
Severe PET/eclampsia
Diabetes mellitus
Rhesus disease
Malpresentation
Cord prolapse
Fetal distress
Multiple pregnancy
Poor obstetric history

Incidence
4–20%

Types
Classical: mid-line uterine incision
Lower segment: transverse or vertical uterine incision in the lower
                          segment

Abdominal incisions
Pfannenstiel
Sub-umbilical mid-line

Complications
Those common to any anaesthetic
Mendelson's syndrome
Haemorrhage
Wound infection
Endometritis
Pulmonary embolism
Respiratory tract infection
Scar rupture in subsequent pregnancies

Primary Post Partum Haemorrhage
Definition: Maternal bleeding in excess of 500 ml
                              occuring within 24 hours of delivery
Note: Serious and potentially lethal
         Blood loss tends to be under-estimated at delivery

Incidence: varies: 3–10%
                              has increased in recent years

Causes:	failure of uterus to contract due to retained products/placenta uterine atony trauma to: uterus cervix vagina perineum
Predisposing factors:	overdistended uterus (eg twins) grand multiparity ('baggy uterus') instrumental delivery use of oxytocics

Management:
Preventive: active management of the third stage using syntometrine and controlled cord traction to deliver the placenta

Treatment of established PPH: set up i.v.i and cross match blood give ergometrine 0.5 mg i.v. (unless contraindicated) transfuse if in doubt and certainly if patient is symptomatic or in hypovolaemic shock

Treatment of specific causes: massage uterus ('rub up a contraction') syntocinon drip bimanual compression of uterus hysterectomy is the last resort

Retained placenta (or part of): remove (under GA)
Tears/lacerations: repair under local/general anaesthesia

Complications death
renal failure
Sheehan's syndrome (rare but famous)
post partum anaemia

The puerperium

Definition: The time taken for the mother to recover from the effects of childbirth and delivery. Note that this does not imply a return to the precise pre-pregnant state. Traditionally, it lasts for anything between 6 weeks to 3 months.

PHYSIOLOGY OF THE PUERPERIUM

The uterus: Bulk reduces by involution following withdrawal of oestrogens:

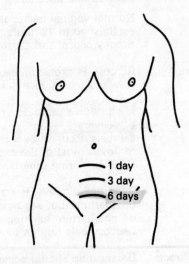

1 day
3 day
6 days

Fig. 43 Uterine involution following delivery; fundal height at 1, 3 and 6 days post-delivery

– by day 1:   18 weeks size
– by day 3:   16 weeks size
– by day 6:   14 weeks size
– by day 10–12:   not palpable
                           abdominally (but note
                           that it never quite
                           returns to its
                           nulliparous size).

Uterine contractions, expelling cast-off debris, give rise to after pains (which are often exacerbated by breast feeding).

Cervix takes on its split parous appearance.

Lochia:

Defined as the uterine discharge following delivery.

Often heavier after breast feeding. Normally lasts for 3–6 weeks:
– first few days — mainly blood
– the next 7–10 days — serosanguinous
– the remaining time till cessation — yellowish.

Consists of red blood cells, white cells, decidua and fibrinous products.

Normal vaginal bacterial flora re-established in 72 hours: includes *E. coli*, *Staphylococci* and *Clostridium welchii*.

Ovarian function:

Returns as prolactin levels fall
New pregnancy rare in less than 6 weeks

Urinary tract:

Micturition should occur within 12 hours of delivery.
Diuresis occuring over the next 2–5 days removes most of the excess fluid retained during pregnancy.

Blood:

Haemoglobin level is stable by 5th day postpartum (but see below for when to do postpartum haemoglobin).
Leucocytosis returns to normal.

Gastrointestinal tract:

Defaecation should occur by day 3 (depending on whether enema given or not).
Constipation is common.

Mental state:	Elation may give way to '5th day blues' (possibly due to hormonal changes).

AIMS OF PUERPERAL CARE

Restoration of optimum maternal health (including prevention, or detection if necessary, of bleeding, sepsis and thrombo-embolism).

Achievement of optimum infant health

Establishment of bonding

Establishment of lactation

Education of the mother

Rapid return of the mother to normal life

ROUTINE PUERPERAL CARE

Observations:	Temperature; pulse and blood pressure Uterine size daily Lochia daily Urine output Bowels Haemoglobin (day 5) (but note that recent evidence suggests day 1 haemoglobin approximates best to 6 week haemoglobin)
Analgesia:	For after pains
Sedation:	If unable to sleep
Perineum:	Removal of sutures not needed provided absorbable sutures used for episiotomy repair Pain relief: air ring analgesics local heat ultrasound ice packs for oedema local creams/foams
General:	Post-natal exercises Attention to diet Psychological support Education in mothercraft

Physio

Infant feeding:

Breast feeding versus bottle feeding: current medical opinion tends to favour breast feeding, but if bottle feeding is intended, suppress lactation early.

Advantages of breast feeding:
- more easily digested by the infant simple, safe and free
- the infants chance of gastrointestinal and possibly other infections is reduced contains the right things in the right amounts
- overfeeding is almost impossible uterine involution is assisted the incidence of subsequent breast carcinoma is reduced if mother less than 20 years
- reduced incidence of eczema in infant

Methods of suppressing lactation:
- bromocriptine
- reduce fluid intake
- provide firm support
- analgesia as required

Discharge:

May be early (48 hours or less) or longer

Advantages of early discharge:
- rapid bed throughput, so allowing increased percentage of hospital deliveries
- reduced risk of maternal/neonatal hospital acquired infection
- some obstetric units are dingy and depressing places
- early discharge is often preferred by the patient

Advantages of longer lying in period:
- mother goes home more rested
- more time is available to educate the mother
- lactation can be better established
- longer relief from the housework
- medical problems developing in the mother or infant after 48 hours are more likely to be noticed

Post-natal visit:	Usually done at 6 weeks, patients usually prefer to visit GP rather than hospital.
Mother:	history of blood loss or pain
	examine weight and blood pressure
	examine breasts: nipples
	masses
	examine pelvic organs: episiotomy for healing
	state of cervix
	uterine size and mobility
	smear test if not done antenatally
	contraception
Infant:	full history especially — feeding
	weight gain
	examination especially — umbilicus
	circumcision if present
	neurological development

PUERPERAL COMPLICATIONS

Puerperal pyrexia

Definition:	Any febrile condition occuring in a woman in whom a temperature of 38°C or more has occurred within 14 days after confinement or miscarriage
Causes:	Genital tract infection
	Urinary tract infection
	Deep vein thrombosis
	Mastitis and breast engorgement
	Respiratory tract infection, especially after anaesthesia
	Other unrelated causes
	Anaemia

SEPSIS

Genital tract infection

Microbiology:	in past: beta-haemolytic Streptococci Gp B were important.

now: anaerobic streptococci (34%)
     staphylococci (23%)
     non-haemolytic Streptococci (19%)
     coliforms (8%)
     remainder (16%)

Any part of genital tract; from vulva to ovary and including the
parametrium may become infected. Usually an ascending
infection.

Features:	malaise
	lower abdominal pain
	offensive lochia
	fever
	tender uterus
Management:	appropriate antibiotic after taking swabs
	and blood cultures (high vaginal and
	cervical swab); give ampicillin ±
	metronidazole until sensitivities known
	analgesia
	hydration and rest
Complications:	sterility
	chronic pelvic inflammatory disease
	broad ligament abscess
	septicaemia
	death

Urinary tract infection
Common, especially following instrumentation.
Often due to *E. coli*

Features:	dysuria, frequency, dull headache
	pyrexia
Investigations:	Haemoglobin, white cell count and
	differential
	mid-stream urine
	high vaginal swab
Treatment:	rest
	analgesia
	high fluid intake
	broad spectrum antibiotic until
	sensitivities known
	mist. pot. cit. for dysuria
	fluid balance chart

Breast infection

Predisposing factors: poor nipple care
breast engorgement

Features: hot red tender area in breast
usually staphylococcal
pyrexia
brawny swelling suggests abscess
formation

Management: if caught early, i.e. less than 48 hr,
antibiotics and suppress lactation
later (or if any suggestion of abscess)
incision and drainage

THROMBOEMBOLISM

Important cause of maternal death   *72-74   76-78 leading cause*

Thrombosis
May occur in leg or pelvic veins

Prevention: early mobilisation, especially after
operative delivery
wear support tights
post-natal exercises
treat anaemia and dehydration

Features: persistent tachycardia, often
disproportionate to any pyrexia
calf pain and tenderness
oedema and swelling of leg
pelvic vein thrombosis (may be
symptomless and signless)

Investigations: Doppler ultrasound
Venogram
Radioisotope studies
Diagnosis is important because of future
implications

Management: raise foot of bed
apply anti-embolism stockings
encourage active movement of legs
heparinise
wafarinise and suppress lactation for 3
months

Embolism
Four grades may be recognised:

Group A: sudden death

Group B: acute dyspnoea with or without evidence
                     of shock

Group C: pleuritic pain and haemoptysis, without
                     circulatory failure

Group D: shortness of breath alone.

Features: call to stool may preceed event
                     giant 'a' wave in jugular venous pulse
                     (blocked pulmonary vasculation)
                     powerful parasternal heave
                     right atrial gallop (triple heart sounds,
                     loudest in the pulmonary area)
                     pleural friction rub in large infarcts.

Investigations: chest X-ray
                     electrocardiogram
                     perfusion scan
                     serum enzymes
                     pulmonary arteriography

Management: acting quickly, on suspicion alone, can
                     save lives: do not waste time doing
                     sophisticated tests unless they are
                     immediately available.
                     restore circulation — cardiac massage
                                             emergency
                                                embolectomy if
                                                available.
                                             thrombolytics (e.g.
                                                urokinase)
                     give oxygen
                     pain relief — Morphine 15 mg i.v.
                     anticoagulate — heparin — 25 000 units
                                                immediately
                                                followed by
                                                25 000 units 6
                                                hourly for 24
                                                hours
                     — wafarinise and suppress lactation

POST PARTUM HAEMORRHAGE

Secondary post partum haemorrhage

Definition: any excess (note no specified volume) genital tract bleeding after 24 hours from delivery.

Causes: first few days — retained products — membranes +/or placenta
blood clots
later infection

Features: fresh vaginal bleeding after lochia has turned brown
tender bulky uterus
os may be open
pyrexia
offensive discharge

Management: resuscitation as needed
high vaginal swab
appropriate antibiotics
surgical exploration (beware of perforating the soft uterus), with evacuation of retained products as appropriate

PSYCHIATRIC COMPLICATIONS

Post-natal depression is common (60%)
   Ranges from '5th day blues' to a severe depressive psychosis

Features: rejection of baby
delusions
confusion

Management: close observation
mild antidepressants
counselling as required

DRUGS AND BREAST FEEDING

Safe	Safety unknown	Unsafe
Heparin	Aminoglycosides	Chloramphenicol
Penicillins	Aspirin	Tetracyclines
Cephalosporins	Beta-blockers	Indomethacin
Codeine	Sulphonamides	Phenylbutazone
Pethidine	Oestrogens (low dose)	Oestrogen (high dose)
Paracetamol	Bronchodilators	Lithium
Methyldopa	Carbimazole	Iodides
Benzodiazepines	Thyroxine	
Phenothiazines	Oral hypoglycaemics	
Tricyclics	Isonaizid	
Digoxin	Ethambutol	
Insulin	Wafarin	
Progesterones		
Antacids		
Bulk laxatives.		

Maternal and perinatal mortality

MATERNAL MORTALITY

Obstetricians in England and Wales have performed their own medical audit in the form of the Confidential Enquires into Maternal Deaths since 1952. (Scotland has been included since 1965.) These enquiries collect detailed informations about maternal deaths over a 3 year period, and thus allow identification of avoidable factors in the causes of death. It has therefore been possible to alter practice so as to considerably reduce maternal mortality. The relative importance of different causes of death has also changed.

An avoidable cause of death was for example identified in obstetric anaesthetic practice in that often inexperienced junior anaesthetists on their own were involved with the cases that went wrong. The British Association of Anaesthetists recommended that two anaesthetists should be present for obstetric anaesthetics, one of whom should be experienced in obstetric anaesthesia. Another report identified an association between artificial rupture of the membranes combined with immediate stimulation of the uterus, resulting in the rare amniotic fluid embolus, which killed 14 women in England and Wales in the triennium 1972–75.

MATERNAL DEATH

Definition: A death occurring during pregnancy, during labour, or as a consequence of pregnancy within *1 year* of the delivery or abortion.

Deaths: 'True' — directly due to pregnancy Associated — due to other causes (i.e. no causal relationship)

Selected facts from the latest report covering 1976–78 (published 1982; HMSO):

227 'true deaths'
200 associated deaths
Maternal mortality rate: 11.9/100 000 total births

Main causes:	Pulmonary embolus — 45 deaths (rising) Hypertensive diseases — 29 deaths (falling) Haemorrhage — 26 deaths (rising) All other causes — 108 deaths
All other causes:	Abortion Cardiac disease in pregnancy Caesarean section Anaesthetic deaths Ruptured uterus Amniotic fluid embolus Ectopic pregnancy Puerperal sepsis Miscellaneous
Associated deaths (for interest only):	Arterial aneurysms Alcoholic disorders Auto-immune diseases Blood diseases: sickle cell anaemia leukaemia Cerebral infarction Diabetes mellitus Encephalitis Epilepsy GI tract disorders Hepatic failure Intracranial haemorrhage Kyphoscoliosis Meningitis Cancer Respiratory disease Renal disease Pituitary infarction

The 'Report on Confidential Enquiries into Maternal Deaths in England and Wales 1976–78', HMSO, London, 1982, makes fascinating reading, and the authors strongly recommend that it is read by undergraduates as an adjunct to the standard testbooks.

PERINATAL MORTALITY AND MORBIDITY

Perinatal mortality is the sum of stillbirths and deaths during the first week of life, and the perinatal mortality rate is the total per 1000 births.

In 1976 the PMR was 18 per 1000 births in England and Wales.

Main causes:	Prematurity (nearly 50% of perinatal deaths occur in preterm infants)
	Intrapartum asphyxia
	Birth trauma
	Malformations
	Hyaline membrane disease
	Pnuemonia
	Unknown (10%)

Associated factors:	Place of residence (S and E best)
	Maternal age (best early 20s)
	Parity (2nd baby best)
	Social class (1 best, 5 worst)
	Poor obstetric history
	Poor antenatal care
	Gestational age
	Birth weight
	PET
	Bleeding before 28 weeks
	Breech delivery
	Forceps delivery
	Prolonged labour
	Precipitate labour

Perinatal morbidity

The incidence of perinatal morbidity is difficult to assess: what criteria are used over what time scale? Which individuals are taken as controls? There is also the difficulty of follow-up.

Perinatal morbidity includes brain damage and the effect of malformations. Although most of the factors affecting the PMR are likely in lesser degrees to influence perinatal morbidity, it is recognised that low social class (and its consequences) are a major factor in increasing perinatal morbidity.

The trend towards smaller families combined with the low PMR (which may have reached its lowest practical level) is resulting in greater emphasis on the quality of obstetric care. Thus it is appropriate to compare not only the mortality rates of different practices, such as forceps delivery and Caesarean section, but also their morbidity. Roughly equal mortalities may mask differences in morbidity. At the end of the day, parents want high quality children, and it is the job of the obstetrician to put a healthy baby in the cot next to a healthy mother.

Index

187